T0209926

ARCTURIAN STAR CHRONICLES

VOLUME THREE

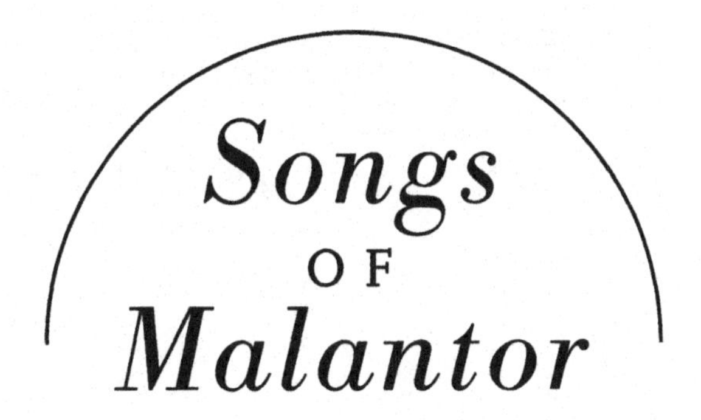

Songs OF *Malantor*

Intergalactic
Seed Messages for
the People of Planet Earth

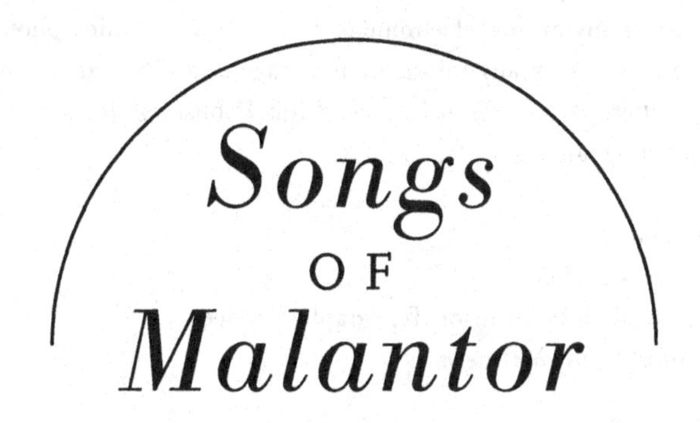

Songs of Malantor

A manual to aid in understanding
matters pertaining to
personal and planetary evolution

Patricia L. Pereira

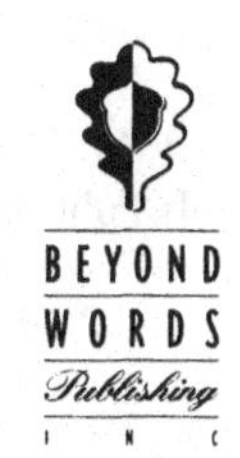

Beyond Words Publishing, Inc.
20827 N.W. Cornell Road, Suite 500
Hillsboro, Oregon 97124-9808
503-531-8700
1-800-284-9673

Editor: Sue Mann
Proofreader: Marvin Moore
Composition: William H. Brunson Typography Services
Managing editor: Kathy Matthews

Printed in the United States of America
Distributed to the book trade by Publishers Group West

Library of Congress Cataloging-in-Publication Data
Pereira, Patricia L.
Songs of Malantor : Intergalactic seed messages for the people of planet earth : a manual to aid in understanding matters pertaining to personal and planetary evolution / Patricia L. Pereira.
p. cm. – (Arcturian star chronicles ; v. 3)
Includes bibliographical references.
ISBN 978-1-885223-70-8 (pbk.)
1. Human-alien encounters. 2. Telepathy. I. Title.
II. Series: Pereira, Patricia L. Arcturian star chronicles ; v. 3.
BF2050.P467 1998
133.9'3–dc21 98-22008
CIP

The corporate mission of Beyond Words Publishing, Inc.:
Inspire to Integrity

In memory of Jeff

Table of Contents

Malantor of Arcturus is a fifth- and sixth-dimensional being of light. His vibrational identity, Malantor, means "creator of melodious lyrics." Malantor is an Arcturian poet and intergalactic counselor-teacher on Earth assignment. He has a masculine vibration, which easily harmonizes with Patricia.

Galactic information in Songs of Malantor, *Volume Three of the Arcturian Star Chronicles, is more complex than information contained in Volume One,* Songs of the Arcturians, *and Volume Two,* Eagles of the New Dawn.

The Song of Malantor

Tranquility is the savior.

Tranquility is the lodge house of the survivors.

Tranquility is the norm of God's Creation.

Tranquility is a state of being worth striving for.

May tranquility fill your loins, may your bones fill with tranquility's vibrant essence. May blessed peace illuminate the contours of your entire body.

May tranquility's perfumed aromas fill the passages of your mind. May your nostrils flare as tranquility's sweet bouquet stimulates your desire, your appetite for God.

Be bold in your spiritual search. Be an adventurer seeking immortal truths. Do not let the wayward glances of others distract you from your Soul's path.

Is there any other delight worth pursuing?

Can any essence fill one to overflowing as do the magnificent robes of God's Creation?

May none other come before you!

Fly as innocently as a bluebird winging into the ecstasy of the future. For it will come to pass that all sorrow will evaporate from the lands of Earth as if a great fog lifted from before your eyes.

Reprinted from Volume Two, *Eagles of the New Dawn.*

Introduction to Malantor

Early December 1987

Patricia, hark to the vibrational hum of your principal guide, Palpae. I have just returned from a sojourn to the Blue Crystal Planet of Arcturus, and I bring with me the gift of another counselor-teacher to accompany your life's journey. This day, the date of your birth celebration, seemed an auspicious time to introduce Malantor. This entity's essence resonations are complementary to yours. Under his excellent tutelage your knowledge of the spiritual nature of the cosmos will continue to grow.

Adonai. The pleasantness of this brief connection will be enhanced as you move forward in the life that will culminate in your return to your starry Arcturian home.

I, Malantor of Arcturus, hail greetings upon you. I introduce self as an intergalactic counselor-teacher who vibrates in accordance with the resonating energies of the

Blue Crystal Planet of the Arcturian star system. I present self in this fashion so you may recognize and acknowledge the essential nature of my being. Know this, Patricia: We will be working as One upon writings of great import.

Patricia, you are one who vibrates as Manitu, spirit keeper. Your essence radiates vibrant colored light. Ever vigilant of the sacredness of the documents you have been entrusted with, you habitually scrutinize them in an attempt to adapt each subtle nuance into the intricate details of your life. Your talents as a telepathic recorder-transmitter escalate. Because we are bonded in service to universal harmony, our mutual purpose will become apparent as my communications unfold.

This being of light, Malantor, has been willingly dispatched to this spatial quadrant at the request of the Regency star council and the Spiritual Hierarchy to aid in establishing various Earth-ascension coordinates. I assume my new assignment in a fervor of ecstatic delight.

Patricia, our communiques will settle into a distinctive style of poetic prose. As our thoughts entwine like vines resting upon an ancient tree, many words will fall upon the pages of your manuscript like sparkles of rain upon a summer lawn. Eventually, our creative efforts will bring renewed hope to many people.

I have been apprised of the spiritual progress evolving humans have made to harmonize their vibrations with Earth as she prepares to journey through the fourth dimension and contemplates emerging into the peaceful realms of the light dimensions. Associated activities unfold upon the starships as entities from the stars move about in wonder as they observe these marvelous events.

As time allows (and we are aware you have precious little), you might place a colored marker on the above lines; they will encourage you to continue your yearning odyssey to the stars in the difficult years ahead. They will serve as a natural focal point as the delicious rhythms of these essays play out.

To continue with our mutual history, Patricia-Manitu, my essence being experiences heightened pleasure as I facilitate coordinating energy patterns within your wandering thoughts. I would awaken your Soul Memories to recall long-forgotten times when you were a sister to Malantor in the days of the Roman Empire. In that life you attempted to create a state of peace and harmony within my then-dispirited self.

I would reawaken you to our Soul connection. Presently, I reside upon the magnificent mother ship, *Marigold–City of Lights*, whose perfumed essence closely resembles your favorite flower.

Before I continue, I will explain the manner in which I recently transmuted a third-dimensional physical body and assumed Arcturian light-energy vibration. Although it is true this is my first mind-aware trip through the webs of energy that catch and hold Earth in her spatial position around the sun, it is not my first residency assignment to this world.

Many aeons ago my being came to experience the human form. However, my spirit body departed this galactic sector prior to the bedeviling situations that currently permeate human affairs.

My final incarnation upon Earth was as a soldier when the legions of Rome stalked the lands. Proudly I supported myself and my family as a warrior, strutting about so that one and all might behold the gleaming eagle emblems emblazoning my Roman uniform. Foolishly ignorant was I that such an arrogant display would fracture the delicate fibers of my spirit's light structures. Thus, as a man young in years, an ignoble death came upon me. Quickly, and somewhat unusually, my spirit body was transferred to another planet under another star; my sleeping spirit found itself caught in the coarse, restrictive energies of a water-based planet. I endured much time sunk in the sticky mire of that dark and dismal world as I remained in the physical confines of a succession of clamlike sea creatures. It was an ugly place, not nearly as pleasant in demeanor as beauteous Earth.

At best it was a gloomy planet, for the seas did not part to absorb morning sunlight for the drawing off of vaporous night air. Recently, however, I was forced into a rapid awakening when star-council members who monitor planetary ascension procedures were dispatched by That Which Guides Universes to summon me to tend to sea urchins' vibrations (the predominant creatures of that unsavory world), for the sunless waters kept my cousins in an agitated, tumultuous state.

As my ancient knowledge resurfaced, my forgotten Soul Memories returned. As I awoke, I called out "Manitu," for I suddenly remembered the name of my revered Soul-sister. Pulled further and further back in time, I recalled the abrupt explosion of our beloved green planet, Cheuel of Arcturus. I retained memories of the wondrous times upon Cheuel when we gamboled and frolicked on her magnificent forests and plains prior to the terrible tragedy.

Careless, careless were we! Suddenly, our spirit lights were flung across the galaxy. We came to land (not willy-nilly, surely, but for the most part firmly planted) upon Cheuel's twin planet—Earth. Here we were granted many opportunities and much time to stoke our fires' karmic embers. Eventually, we accepted our fate and settled down to mesh our spirits with Earth's bountiful soils. Thus we began the recycling process of multilayered incarnate lives.

Now here comes Malantor, presenting his essence self (as your visionary mind perceives) as an airy fifth- and sixth-degree entity formed of light. Absorbed in Love-Light energy, I presently function within the naturally sweet tonations of the higher-magnitude rhythms as an integrated member of the Arcturian Council of Elders. It is a meritorious honor to find my I Amness existing as One with beings of light who serve Divine Intelligence upon the Regency star council.

At long last, Malantor's I Amness is robed in starlight energy; but this did not occur until my Soul struggles were complete and I was granted permission to transmute physical form to spiritual form. Through countless lifetimes, through untold incarnations, I journeyed through the lower dimensions. Nevertheless, I have ascended to harmoniously blend my Soul's simple yet intricate energies with those of the Arcturian light worlds.

Regarding the title description of a manitu: The energy identity characteristic of a manitu, or spirit keeper, was laid down as a vibrational setting on Earth through energies widely dispersed throughout the North American continent via the wise teachings of people who were indigenous to that world sector. Manitu is a symbolic reference title or job description bestowed by the Spiritual Hierarchy upon humans who are entrusted with maintaining nature's harmonies. Manitus hold Earth's best interests in high regard, for they are careful monitors of the stability of the planetary grids. Manitus protect and shield Earth with waves of passionate love that radiate transformative heat from the center of their heart cores. Essentially, manitu force-field energy is easily achieved. The vibrational title *manitu* is a resource identification we use to discern an individual's higher purpose from that of others, such as those who are healers of disease or mental distress.

Earth, in these, the latter days of her third-dimensional placement, is in dire need of her spirit keepers, for manitus are frontline planetary energy defenders. During these accelerated times, manitus greatly assist the star travelers as we work together to transform Earth's physical structures to light.

It is becoming commonplace for humans to want to serve Spirit in some profound way. The combined energies exuded by these dedicated men and women represent Genesis of One merging into Being. As groups of humans focus their intention upon a common goal, such as Earth-healing meditations, their united thoughts fuse into a solid mass of transformative supercharged energy. Many marvelous humans who routinely participate in Earth-healing practices are purposefully interacting with extraterrestrial beings of light.

We deem those who are awakening to Soul service as esteemed warriors of light, as eagles of the new dawn. The numbers volunteering to harmonize their lives with the evolving Earth rhythms escalate daily. Now we no longer ride aboard our rainbow-hued ships virtually ignored by humans.

Millennia ago, even in millions of years, fertile Earth was abundantly planted with the Soul-essence energies of extraterrestrial beings from several star systems, such as the Pleiades, Arcturus, Orion, and Sirius. Ancient in Soul, these starseeds are beginning to resemble lush, lovely fruit: Many are ripe for harvesting. As they mature, we will gently gather their delicate blooms and set them upon a course of life-purpose fulfillment. Long encased in shells of dormant forgetfulness and subjected to torturous centuries of indignant death-life recycling, these stalwart beings, despite their difficulties, are managing to awaken. One fine day, when their life journeys are complete, the children of the stars will mount the steps of the space chariots and, at long last, joyfully return to their starry homes.

Stay acutely aware during these heightened years, for a day will dawn when an evolved sun spills its magnificent rays upon Earth's graceful hills. On that day, brilliant-hued starships will descend and entities representing the Regency star council will present themselves for your inspection, after which a glorious celebration will commence. On that day, our precious fledglings, our eagles in Oneness with the crew of intergalactic starships, will fly!

I, Malantor, am a Soul brother to all humans. My home world is the Blue Crystal Planet of the Arcturian star system. Ambassador Palpae, Patricia's primary contact, and myself are members of the Council of Arcturian Elders. As Patricia's energy aligns in expansive agreement with fifth- and sixth-dimensional Arcturians, our mutual thought resonations, silent sound set in motion, create a unique blending of light particles, solar communication, the universal language of the many suns.

Ring the holy bells in ecstatic song, for now is the most sacred time in all Earth's history. Hark! May a joyous sound emanate from the depths of your hearts. This is an auspicious occasion to augment the teachings of He Who Yet Roams Earth, the Christ Essence. Despite these wondrous times, many are enmeshed in the rigors of ignoble suffering, the likes of which never seem to end. No sooner do they lay aside one distressful emotion than another appears to take its place, and what they thought was finished suddenly resurfaces. As we critically observe humans, we realize that the statistical probability of their single-handedly resolving that which greatly torments them will prove impossible without the cooperative assistance of benevolent beings who have pledged themselves in service to Omnipotent Light.

Although life may appear to have been harsher for preindustrial people in terms of creature comforts and daily proximity to death, from our starships it would appear little has changed. Perhaps the abundance and variety of foodstuffs is greater and the textiles you weave your garments from much softer. Nevertheless, the overall intensity of suffering and pain is much greater and more widespread. A constant barrage of negative, agitation-producing information exuded by the media is extremely detrimental to the psyche. The majority of the population are on the verge of plunging into a morass of profound, hopeless despair.

You who are awakening to the presence of a variety of cosmic intelligences visiting Earth are urged to strengthen yourselves for the difficult years that lie ahead. Avoid falling into a trap of discouragement. Focus your thoughts upon the brilliant promises of the newly birthing century. Be inspired to spiritually self-determine. Approach your daily activities with the intention of preparing for eventual ascension into bodies of refined light.

Adonai.

Introduction to the Oneness of Being That Is Malantor-Patricia

To address logical difficulties posed by your rational mind, Patricia: As you know, we offer alternative methods to process thought. It is important for you to assimilate our teaching that the energy conduit representative of Malantor-Patricia is one and the same (as is Palpae-Patricia), although from your human perspective we are separate entities. The vibrational Soul essence Malantor, who hails from the Blue Crystal Planet of the Arcturian star system, is resonation sensitive to light-quality vibrations that comply with the rosy Arcturian sun. Soul-Self Malantor also integrates in a rather unique fashion with Earth and her sun, Sol, via the telepathic starseed modality known as Patricia or Manitu. Malantor, however, dwells in a finer-dimensional octave pitch—as you are "lower-scale C" compared to my "higher-scale C."

Patricia, as you learn to encompass your emotional heart-mind thoughts with your brain's compartmentalized mental processing, the Soul-Self of this multiple entity in

Oneness that is we-I will become an essential component of your daily life. Malantor-Patricia exists simultaneously as a Soul-Self entity that inhabits many multilevel planes in at least two star systems simultaneously. We are actually many beings arising from a same cell or Soul embryo at the time of Creation's "beginning" (an inaccurate term limited to the restrictions of third-dimensional cosmic comprehension).

Though we may express ourselves as a part of this and a part of that, at Soul level the experience is that of one being. We-I are incapable of being divided or separated. We-I have never been so, nor ever will we be. Entity Malantor-Patricia may better be described by one vibrational identification, perhaps as Patriciamalantor or Malantorpatricia, it matters not.

We urge you, Patricia, to a fuller, richer comprehension of the thought energies that weave in and out of your conscious mind. Not only are you in perpetual Soul Oneness with Malantor of Arcturus, but also you are with Palpae of Arcturus as well as with many other individuals in Oneness who reside at many multilevel dimensions. What is herein addressed as a quivering being of delight we call Patricia of Earth is, in reality, identical Soul essence with many beings from many universes.

"How can this be?" your skeptical mind queries.

It is simply illustrated thusly:

I am placing before your third eye a picture of a bright light, as if it were issuing forth from a stationary lamp. Now I place a thin slice of paper in the middle of the bulb so it appears that the light has separated into two halves. In reality, only one light source exists. If you can use this simple analogy to depict the creation and division of a Soul cell, you may get some glimmering of what is meant.

Take one more step in this pictorial essay. Continue to see the strip of paper lying in the middle of the bulb. Notice that two beams of light are generated. The one that tracks to the right illuminates a wall, for to illuminate the right wall is the purpose of that beam. The other beam tracks to the left and shines its brilliance upon a shaded window, for to illuminate a darkened window is the purpose of the left beam. As these two functions are accomplished, the whole purpose of the lamp's existence is served, for its greater purpose is to illuminate every area of the room. This is also Creator's purpose for forming Soul: to illuminate the contours of the void in which unlimited space is contained.

The right beam and the left beam are two parts of an identical whole. If they are one and the same, how can they be divided? Separation is an illusion, an external quality of Earth life. Its component textures have no bearing on the eternal inner Soul—that which knows itself as One.

That which is you-I, Patricia, resembles an exquisite Greek statue in that we are perfected in a manner modern art no longer pursues, but its marbled contours are still widely appreciated. Indeed, your awakening Soul Memories stand as a silent tribute to another age, another place in spatial time. That which you have dreamed since you were a wee babe is to reunite self as Essence of Soul.

That purpose is our mutual purpose, and as such we serve Divine Creator. It is our Soul's purpose to gather and balance light so that one side of our being hums in poetic mastery with the other side of our being as we jot down tidbits with which to entice humans to join the galactic chorus in one ecstatic song.

This writing represents only a minor function of our Soul's greater purpose, but it is enough to share with you in these opening remarks. We will use our I Amness in a tantalizing way to tease others into daring to know themselves from a higher reality.

Patricia, do not be intimidated when asking spiritual beings questions that are pertinent to your daily life. It is your right to seek knowledge on any level that is meaningful to you, particularly as you have opted to struggle for a clearer picture of the universe and its laws.

That is enough for today, Patricia-Manitu. Adjourn now and assume a more comfortable position. You can leave for another day the wanderings of your fingertips over your computer keyboard as you express your delight in communicating telepathically with Malantor of Arcturus.

Adonai.

About Patricia

Patricia has requested Malantor's assistance in explaining why she was selected by the Arcturians and the star councils to interact with them as a transdimensional telepath.

Let it please Malantor to begin. This one, Patricia, we ask you to understand, is dedicated to serving Earth in cooperative alliance with other humans and animals who care for their world as catalytic evolutionary enhancers, one of many details pertaining to multispecies and planetary ascension. It is further stated that most humans would deem this woman (and others like her) a silly dreamer, a person of minute import with no valid point of view as to the true substance of reality. Yet in the eyes of fifth- and sixth-dimensional extraterrestrials, her heart, mind, and intent to serve Earth's creatures brightly shine.

It was requested of Patricia-Manitu (as we commonly address her) in the summer of 1987 to ride as One with the telepathic minds of Arcturian beings of light who monitor

Earth from multidimensional starships. Simultaneously, we presented her with several major challenges and very little time to make her decisions. We asked that she assume the responsibility of preparing a collection of transdimensional information seed packets. We advised her that if she heeded our summons, she would step off the path her life currently embraced and that she passionately loved, one that greatly favored her temperament: her work to support habitats for wolves. She willingly rearranged her priorities and eagerly placed herself under the tutelage of her Arcturian advisors. Thus, she accepted the great burden we thrust upon her.

Responding to our summons with barely a backward glance, Patricia stored all she loved into a basket of past memories and set forth upon her new mission from transition base Boise, Idaho. Journeying a short day's distance, she arrived at the edge of a region of rarefied vortex energies where the city of Spoke-ane, Washington, somewhat precariously perches upon the northwest grid of the North American continent. Settling into her new assignment in earnest, she began the task of lovingly recording the messages her extraworld colleagues were sending her.

On a winter's night in the same year, Malantor initiated thought-link with Patricia-Manitu. Great was our Soul joy as the Oneness of our beings, long lost to each other, was reestablished.

We who voyage to Earth from the Arcturian planetary cluster to serve the Christ Essence select individuals to assist us who generally appear of little consequence to other humans. Men and women who willingly thought-connect with ultradimensional beings emit waves of high-intensity energy ideal for evolutionary healing procedures and for incorporating light into Earth's body.

Assuredly, Patricia's natural abilities to telepathically focus upon Earth's enhancing vibrations bear little resemblance to those that would qualify her as a candidate for employment in corporate megabusyness. Nevertheless, Patricia's primary assets are her dedication to a spiritual cause she barely understands and her drive to manifest Soul purpose—which burns within her like an all-consuming flame.

Patricia, a woman of middle years, is burdened with a mystically oriented mind and a perpetual hunger for spiritual knowledge. When she was a child, she began flinging wild, yearning petitions into the ethers. Unabashedly she would challenge the starships to come down to her. "Help us! Help us!" she would cry into the night. Inevitably, her passionate pleas became caught in the finely meshed nets of the space chariots' crystalline thought monitors. There they were recorded and stored until the moment of her precoded awakening. Although she has gained much insight into the nature of the cosmos, she still wonders about many things and often feels suspended between two worlds—Earth's rocky crust and the Arcturian starships she longs to board. This perplexing state of affairs is quite common to awakening starseeds. We predict that before the days of this century draw to a close, humans who have committed themselves in service by integrating Source Energy into all they think, say, and do will find themselves entangled in many situations in which their motives and belief systems are greatly misunderstood.

Because Patricia's experiences parallel those of other starseeds, ponder upon the implications and significance of these data for yourself. We suggest you consider each essay a personal treasure we carefully designed to enhance the quality of your life.

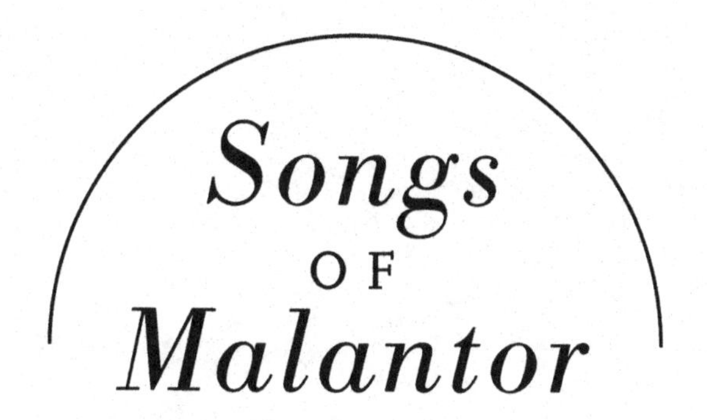
Songs
OF
Malantor

Regarding Human Ability to Adapt to Cosmic Evolutionary Changes

You must create a dynamic plan of action geared toward permanent change before you can expect to effectively alter habitual patterns of behavior. To be successful in such a project, you must first thoroughly examine and modify all your entrenched and outmoded physical, emotional, mental, and spiritual attitudes. When you resolve to surrender peacefully to your Soul's great plan for incarnating in a physical body—an essential step in the awakening process—you will become determined to activate spiritually.

To aspire to the achievement of cosmic enlightenment is a magnificent endeavor. An enterprise of this magnitude requires that galactic aspirants learn to carefully monitor and discern soft influxes of thought that run through the depths of their minds like gentle, flowing rivers. Overcome the habit of murky thought processing, a disagreeable tendency of industrialized society to categorize sudden outbursts of intuitive clarity as suspicious forms of paranormal phenomena. It is a common practice among most humans to virtually ignore any telepathically transmitted information that filters into their brains, for they fear being led down blind alleys. Although they are an essentially intelligent species, in their desire to maintain separation they have developed the attitude that thought-blending is belittling, intrusive, dangerous, and an insubstantial means of communication. As a result, they move through their lives in a semipermanent state of cosmic blindness, their view of other dimensions effectively blocked by a barrage of narrow-minded, dogmatic, linear-structured beliefs. Those who refuse to embrace a multi-level universal viewpoint radically sever their ties with their greater galactic family.

It is not unusual for Earth people to feel encased in a shell of inescapable grief, fear, and anger, with little comprehension regarding the underlying reasons for their difficulties. They display the basic human need to assure themselves that there are rational explanations for their troubles. Because they are fundamentally sensitive and tender, in their anguish they seek self-other consolation and tidy, culturally acceptable justification for intense states of emotional and mental disability. A common practice assigns popular psychological phrases, such as "job situational stress syndrome," to explain chronic and acute discomfort.

From our vantage points, we observe that your awakening hearts are stirred more by the sweet callings of the future than by the sorrowful renditions of the past. Brilliant stanzas and exquisite refrains originating from beings who live upon worlds of refined resonation herald the opening of a new dawn age. Earth Mother hums with anticipation that she, too, will have a graceful journey into the light realms. Although the future beckons like a tantalizing view from around a distant corner, the dawn of each new day brings heightened awareness of the sweetness of the coming age.

Your higher Selves know that wondrous events are unfolding. Still, the majority tenaciously cling to the status quo and to scientifically acceptable explanations of paranormal mysteries. Humans who are steeped in mental-intellectual traditions generally reject outright any inward urgings to evolve spiritually. Certainly, they fail to pay diligent attention to our somewhat illusive will-o'-the-wisp exhortations to mature cosmically. Nevertheless, their Soul-Selves are well aware that extraterrestrial beings who inhabit magnificent worlds of celestial light are in residence Earthside.

Unwittingly, long ago humanity took certain, now well-established playmates to their bosoms, dark entities who delighted in introducing their particularly rowdy companions to humans: fear of death and its inevitable twin fear of life. Surely, it is an anomaly that Love-loving humanity became so entranced with the shiny garb that destructive-prone beings wear and their noisy, troublesome ways. Understand, any being who sucks at and saps your vitality and demands your precious energy does not represent Love-Light.

Ponder deeply upon our extrasolar musings and redefine fear's energies within the dictionary of your perceptual understanding. Mull on these essays like a puppy with a fresh bone. Demonstrate an act of budding wisdom and dissipate the energies of inward negativity. Carefully analyze any remaining surges of attraction you have for fear's destructive ways. Launch yourselves upon a solid, well-defined campaign to permanently eradicate humanity's ancient enemies. Attack fear at its roots with its oppositional foe, all-inclusive Love. Unconditional Love, or cosmic substance, has the capacity to be used as building material for physical manifestation. Love is the foundation from which stars are formed. Love is the mortal adversary of entities who honor fear's ways. It is as impossible for fear-entrenched beings to coexist within a force field of applied unconditional Love as it is for shadows to remain when showered with radiant light.

Clear away any foggy inward vision that limits your perceptions to third-dimensional sight. Imagine yourself and your grand planet, Lady Earth, situated within another plane of existence, living in sweet accord with delightful companions, the residents of fifth- and sixth-vibratory light spectrums. Be aware in every fiber of your being that Earth is inexorably gravitating toward a new dawn future, and she daily enhances and refines the pitch of her celestial song.

Allow the pages of this book to open spontaneously. As you read, know that its phrases and paragraphs are duplicated in the creative endeavors of many writers, composers, artists, and cinematic adventurers. Telepathed communications generated by star-field beings are visually and audibly penetrating into the far corners of the planet.

Their rhythms and lyrics essentially merge as One, though the melodies' many nuances may appear to be composed of a wide variety of features. The underlying theme of all these works is of species and planetary evolution. Awakening humans are attempting to implement the teachings as life-focused material, although the masses persist in limiting themselves to the study of separatism common to humans who oppose the Law of One as applicable to human society.

Through many physical incarnations you have meandered somewhat forlornly down one well-trod highway. From life to life, in a somewhat distracted manner, you have jostled back and forth attempting to maneuver through the mazelike recycling indigenous to Souls whose spirits are tied to Earth's third-dimensional energies. At long last your lonely road has come to a major fork. Two well-marked signs clearly indicate a choice. The branch to the right resembles a path of golden bricks, the preferred route of those who vibrate Love's energies. It is a narrow causeway requiring close and constant monitoring to safely navigate. Those who successfully traverse Love's course will eventually find themselves bathed in the brilliant light of a refreshed sun where angels gather to welcome them Home.

The leftward road is a downward-sloping path. Although at first glance it would seem easier to traverse, it is gloomy and bathed in subtly progressing shadows emanating little or no God Light or Love. In those dreadful lands the Dark Lords await the unwary, attempting to trap them in the fear-drenched caverns of the nether worlds.

Search diligently for what you have lost! Oil those rusty hinges that sequester your hungry mind behind the opening doorways of your Soul. To do so, you must first acknowledge that you have lost something immeasurably precious.

The thoroughfare to Cosmic Home is not cumbersome and is easier to travel than most have been taught to believe. Its signposts are not obscurely marked. Home's flowered portals reside on the avenue of unconditional Love.

Be an intrepid explorer, one who is never daunted. Have the courage to delve into and explore that mysterious being—your true Self. Humanity's great spiritual masters have always taught that the way Home is an inward journey. To begin, you must be solid and very clear in knowing that you are and have always been God's beloved child. You must believe that you are precious, unique, and exquisitely beautiful. You must be explicitly and constantly true to yourself. In times of torment, tragedy, and despair you must stay spiritually focused. Remember, all situations you find yourself in are adapted by your Soul as a means for accelerated growth.

We urge you to be quite daring in exploring the recesses of your inner being. Adventure forth with a heroic attitude. Be as passionate in your drive to uncover the mysteries of your unknown Self as are the intrepid men and women who prowl Earth's polar regions, who probe the oceanic depths, and who succumb to the enchanting lure of the stars. Strive to emulate the truly courageous—those humans who burn with an unquenchable desire to (re)discover their higher Selves, indeed a trek of considerable personal consequence.

Do not allow grief or spiritual laziness to deflect you from embarking upon life's most worthy endeavor. With great fanfare we suggest it is more than time for you to become alert, for something quite profound is happening all around you.

Search! Search! For your lost Self, search!

The I Amness of Malantor of Arcturus is pledged in service to the great brotherhoods of the solar core. In your solar system, the Arcturian contingency of the Intergalactic Brotherhood of Light has established operations upon Saturn. The Supreme Hierarchical Council for Planetary Ascension, System Sol, oversees all interplanetary and intergalactic "business matters" in this sun sector. Beings of light in residence Sol system are multispecies, multigalactic, and multiuniversal; many Earth people have long been designated members of the Regency star council.

May this essay's overtones resonate as high truth within the emotional fabric of your innermost being.

Salud, awakening starseeds!

Adonai.

The Futility of War and Humanity's Spiritual Resistance

Historically, humans have conspired with certain dark entities whose main interest is to surely (albeit gradually) deflect both individuals and the people as a whole from fulfilling what is best defined as Soul's greater purpose. Though their physical anatomy is built upon elements of spiritual or Love-Light properties, humans' tendency is to respond to their planetary environment in a manner that draws shadowy emanations from the lower-astral regions onto Earth planes. Humans radiate disturbed energies with corresponding behavioral patterns, and the consequences, which are based on fear-driven emotions, are sadly regarded as life's norm. Therefore, a situation has transpired whereby the majority suffer from a general malnourishment of their spiritual bodies. Much unhappiness and misery have resulted from humanity's unfortunate relationship with the Dark Lords.

Through time, the predominant philosophical underpinning of human society has been centered around a construct-destruct system of beliefs whose roots are embedded in ego-inflating, self-involved, greed-oriented, prideful eccentricity. Though a fairly intelligent and loving species, humanity's heroic myths ironically revolve around traditions steeped in violence and war. Hostile aggression, secret political pacts, and a stockpiling of armaments is deemed essential for even the most idealistic nation, no matter how compelling and honorable the impulse that motivated the country's founders.

On the surface it would appear that humanity's emotional makeup contains an overwhelming inclination to twist and turn Creation's base matter, Love-Light, until its natural radiance is warped to reflect fear's unruly countenance. Paradoxically, coexisting with this unfortunate state of affairs is humans' innate knowledge of and yearning for Utopia's peaceful abode.

From the narrow focus of a generally terrorized species, the manufacture and hoarding of atrocious weapons by society's most powerful governments may appear to be reasonable and sane. What is not generally understood is the dire spiritual ramifications of such behavior. Initially radiating skyward, energies from acts of fear-driven aggression return to cascade upon Earth like nuclear fallout. Bits and clumps of dark debris rain from the sky. Residue in the form of negative-charged energies is real, a situation that originates with and molds itself by shadowy thoughts that, in waves, stream from the sleeping minds of the planet's least cosmically alert citizens.

Seeking to receive pity from and simultaneously discover a means by which they might negotiate a position of cause-justification with Most High God, individuals presiding over humanity's governing, economic, and religious institutions have slid upon hard times. They seem completely unwilling to acknowledge that aggressive acts perpetrated upon others do not meet the standards of God-approved Universal Law, which is based upon energies of unconditional Love.

Universal Law is not generally understood by humanity. The force of the law's clauses have degenerated until only the most spiritually astute and Love-motivated individuals routinely put them into practice. Consequently, those who use the Law of Free Will to manipulate cosmic energy, to exercise it when, if, and how they choose, subject themselves to the rhythms of harmonious balance, the Law of Cause and Effect. Willing participants in war—even when conscripted under military laws designed by their governing officials—inadvertently cast themselves upon a course whose journey may find them swimming through muddy waters from life to life until enough cosmic time has passed for their accumulated karma to receive a thorough scrubbing.

Intentionally projecting hateful thoughts toward others in a real sense constitutes acts of aggressive behavior. Unwittingly, those transmitting such thoughts encapsulate themselves in spirals of karmic energies that wind around their essences like cocoons. Once set in motion, these energies will continue to swirl until such time as their potency is dissipated by an equal infusion of Love-Light energy.

This law—to Love one another—is the paramount teaching! Love is the purifying force before which all negativity dissolves, not only for the edification of humanity but equally so for the multitudes of life forms that exist throughout the many universes.

The bulk of humanity continues to ignore the fundamental principles of Universal Law. The ramifications of such behavior have subjected humans to the difficulties that have historically plagued them.

Seeded as galactic stock, long ago humans chose to deliberately cut the ties that bound them to the Memories of their star ancestry. Thereafter, assuming they were alone in the universe, they began to nourish their increasingly ill-defined, species-oriented egos by falling into a self-induced spiritual coma. Only marginally conscious, they began to believe that human law is superior to Supreme Law, which served only to separate them further and denied them access to the luscious fruits that are served upon the star councils' crystalline tables.

Regardless of your persistence in ignoring our presence, we have remained here to watch over you as best we may, though the Law of Noninterference limits us, particularly through history's harshest periods.

Now, in these latter years of the twentieth century, the bravest of the brave are beginning to reconsider their life priorities. Many are establishing conscious, direct telepathic communication with multidimensional beings of light. Endeavoring to evolve, spiritual pioneers have begun to explore the fertile lands of their innermost selves. Their efforts are effectively redefining the golden wisdom of ancient Earth-loving traditions. Their work is substantially eroding the remaining vestiges of an illusive veil that has long separated humanity from other planes of existence.

Both overt and subtle rhythms exude from a third-dimensional being's auric body, energies so profound that only those who have mastered God-realization can even begin to assess the ramifications of any act or thought let loose upon the planet. However, ordinary people who diligently tend to matters pertinent to their personal spiritual evolution, leaving those things that influence the lives of others to others, are apt to find themselves walking the corridors of magnificent starships in the dawning years of the twenty-first century. In previous volumes we have stated the primary provisions that must be met before humanity's signature can be placed upon the contract that will adopt you individually and collectively into the greater galactic community.

Commitment to self-evolution is in order. Activated humans are swiftly becoming aware that they are in telepathic contact with celestial beings. Humans exemplifying growth qualities are becoming increasingly proficient at exuding energies that enhance Earth-healing procedures in cooperation with members of their galactic family, working in harmonic unison to propel Earth into the comforting arms of higher-octave resonations.

Stalling tactics are a predominant characteristic of the general population when faced with the necessity for massive change. To avoid that which is quickly becoming third-dimensionally obvious, their favorite ploy is to debunk all harbingers of extraterrestrial information as charlatans. This naturally causes starseeds much personal grief, although they have been challenged to serve as soldiers of light in the greatest battle Earth has ever known. Nevertheless, they courageously shoulder their celestial assignments to gently and lovingly break down the barricades of human resistance. They are endeavoring, as best they might, to encourage others to put the elements of all spiritual teachings into daily practice. We know these intrepid beings as sky warriors, eagles of the new dawn. We are aware that their primary weapons are Love, courage, trust, and faith.

This is a composition of a being in Oneness: Malantor of Arcturus and Patricia of Earth. All data generated by the entity in Oneness, Malantor-Patricia, may be considered as a cocreative composition, filed and handled as such. The input of Malantor-Patricia will add a certain poetic clarity to the writings of the self-purifying being we call Manitu in honor of the work she performs, a woman whom friends and family know as Patricia. She resides in an aging human woman's body upon the third planet of the sun Sol. Like many, for several years her light-body has been undergoing a process of cellular transformation. We are preparing her for the moment she will reconnect with her Arcturian family aboard the starships. Like the majority who are awakening to greater purpose, she is consumed with desire to serve her planet and her people. Counted as one among many pioneers of the new dawn, Manitu and those like her are stalwartly engaged in various degrees of personal mental, emotional, physical, and spiritual struggle.

Peace be yours to contemplate, brothers and sisters. Indicate your growing maturity by considering peace in its fullest meaning, for the energies of peace are filed under the label Love-Light. The elemental desire of the energy of peace is to propel her loving components into realms where light shines eternal.

Telepathy, Starships, Challenger, *and the Making of Heroes*

Those who endeavor to quiet the incessant chattering of their computerlike brains are becoming adept at listening to the soft whispers that echo through the substrates of their intuitive minds. You who are learning to surrender to silence are beginning to experience the spontaneous blending of multilayered thought. As humans awaken, a pathway into their pituitary glands opens, making it possible for them to receive our solar-amplified thoughts. We routinely project our thoughts through portal grids located within the sun to strengthen our multidimensional vibration waves before transferring them to telepathic novices. In the pituitary, extraworld solar-enhanced transmissions undergo an energy exchange that transforms them into language, musical notes, or other symbols.

Located in the midbrain, the pituitary's primary communication function is to define image sequences in

Author's note: The *Challenger* shuttle was the ill-fated NASA flight, with a U.S. schoolteacher aboard, that exploded on takeoff in 1987.

recognizable patterns consistent with the individual's tendencies for creative expression. Flowing like a meandering river, telepathic thought then moves into the pineal gland, or third eye, where it gives birth to enhanced visionary pictures.

To novices, receiving transdimensional communications initially plunges them into confusion. In the beginning their sense of reality turns topsy-turvy, as though they were peering at the world through opaque glasses. We recommend routine meditation focused on centering and balancing to help offset these unsettling sensations.

Meditation is a powerful tool. It activates mechanisms within the brain that are necessary for optimal telepathic exchange. Consistent meditators accumulate an extra reserve of cosmic light that naturally insulates them from cacophonous intrusions and disruptive, energy-draining individuals. Silence is easily accessed. Stillness is achieved through routine meditation. Thought-alert individuals eventually come to the realization that they are in continuous contact with beings who dwell in subtler realms of existence.

The intuitive subconscious mind as well as the superconscious Soul mind are consciously accessible through hyper-aware meditation. As a spiritual being having a human experience, you are firmly attached to Source Mind by a cord of brilliant light that ascends up and out your spine through your crown chakra. As you move into deep meditation, Divine Light substance disperses naturally throughout your body with a resultant multiorgan vibrational upgrading of cellular tissue. This is observable in the etheric as bursts of cosmic light flowing through your chakras. From our viewpoint it appears as if twinkling stars were illuminating the deepest, darkest regions of space.

Fields of intuitive clarity are accessed by individuals who consistently seek meditative alignment with the whispering hums that steadily emanate from celestial core. As you make time in your life for periods of quiet contemplation, you will initiate direct access to the angelic realms, to your spiritual mentor guides, and to beings of light who reside aboard extrastellar starships. Love-based thought forms that rise slowly and persistently from deep within your opening heart-mind are your personal ticket to climb on board.

Though they are constantly transmitting, those who remain stubbornly opposed to the receptive telepathic experience view incoming visionary data as weird, dreamlike, hallucinatory. An addictive fondness for incessant chatter drowns out any real connection the majority have with Universal Mind. Their closed-minded brains habitually transform information originating from Cosmic Intelligence into extremely narrow, often negative, unyielding notions of internal and external reality.

On a more cheerful note, intuitive-minded individuals are becoming increasingly adept at accessing silent-state thought. They are learning to immediately tune in when waves of finely pulsing energy flow through their awakening minds. The spiritually awakening are taking their initial steps as consciously aware telepaths—a true encounter of the fourth kind: personal, direct communication with multidimensional beings of light.

As authentic as the accouterments of your home are the disks of flashing light that humans refer to as UFOs. Propellants for operating starships over the celestial roads are a combination of pure refined essences: delicately hued whirling lights, reverberations of softly singing crystals, and brief, aromatic whiffs that arise from rose-tinged spatial grids. Starship fuel is sparked by focused thought.

Space roads are weblike grids of etheric light that crisscross space. Starship design is similar to the makeup of the spatial grids. That is, designers of starships convert light (Love manifested), sound (Aum or Ohm), and smell (essence of space roses, perfumed essence of pure light) into manifest form. Space grids are precursors of cosmic clouds, ribbons of Divine Light and Sound that eventually give birth to suns.

Mimicking the spiraling helix of the genetic matrix, starships soar upward and downward, forward and backward, spinning like tops as the crystalline drive shafts refine the vessels' integral hum. Blending their minds as One, starship personnel create the catalysts that set starships in motion and plot their courses over the delicately humming webs. Volatile fuels or nuclear fission are not necessary. The pulsing rhythm of our thoughts merged with elemental ingredients of the universal hum are quite sufficient to instantly achieve enough thrust to propel us to our destinations. Those who volunteer to maneuver starships over the grids use their thought projections to sustain vibrational heat generated through the drive shafts.

From Earth to Saturn, as quick as the blink of an eye is the rate of speed starships use. Arcturus to Sol, Sol to

Sirius, as it is thought it is achieved. It is not necessary to place our beings into artificial states of suspended animation for centuries. Gaily, playfully, instantaneously we hop from star field to star field and from planet to planet. We live like innocent, carefree children running through meadows of sun-drenched clover.

How we admire the courageous trailblazing of Earth's pioneering astronauts, brave men and women who strap their delicate bodies into rocket-shaped cans filled with tightly compacted explosives. These dauntless beings hurtle into the sky with such force, with gyrations so strong, that the skin of their faces is pulled to the back of their scalps. We view these activities with much alarm. The discomfort these intrepid individuals endure as they are launched into space, the dangers they face, and the anxiety they undergo elicit much compassion from our beings.

The spirit of *Challenger*'s mission will not soon fade from human memory, though she exploded on her innovative flight and plunged crew and cargo into the ocean. The reverberations of the *Challenger* tragedy will long echo in the hearts and minds of those she left behind. It may soften your sorrow to understand that her gallant crew have had their wishes granted. The dream they held in common has come true. Awestruck as delighted children, the liberated spirits of *Challenger*'s marvelous men and women were set free to navigate the star clusters at will. Exiting physical life, their spirit bodies gained instantaneous access to the rainbow-hued hallways of light-dimension starships. Their passion and bravery earned them the right to enjoy full starship privileges. With much personal pleasure and esteem we welcomed them aboard as our companions in exploring the many wonders of the celestial hum.

Do not deplete your energy mourning the men and women of *Challenger*. Comprehend their status from an expanded point of view. *Challenger*'s heroic crew sacrificed their physical lives to bring an enlightened perspective to the greater human family. The symbolism of their fiery "deaths" was meant to point out to even the least astute that humanity will not be allowed access to the peaceful star grids by journeying in what is essentially a bomb—for the prime purpose of a bomb is, of course, to explode: *BOOM! POOF!*

The life-ending, spirit-becoming event that transformed the *Challenger* crew from physical mass to light essence was purposefully initiated by Earth's Spiritual Hierarchy in accordance with each astronaut's Soul mission parameters. The intention behind the "catastrophe" was to shock a people struggling in the dark night of spiritual chaos into greater awareness. It is unfortunate, however, that the brilliant sacrifice of the *Challenger* crew, which was intended to shine like a mirror held high for the edification of its human counterparts, essentially reflected upon the blank faces of a cosmically imperceptive people.

The brave men and women of *Challenger* are the legitimate heroes and heroines of a heroless age. These courageous souls dared to live their dreams. They dared to fulfill a purpose that far outstripped the routine confinements of their everyday lives. Visionary and inspired, they were motivated to strive for supreme achievement no matter the personal cost. The strength of their mutual resolve magnifies the harmony that exists whenever a people cooperatively unify to manifest their Souls' greater purpose.

Do not gossip about any minute transgressions you may have heard that appear to have tarnished the lives and relationships of the *Challenger* astronauts. Instead, may the beauty of their sacrifice serve as a spark to ignite admiration for their valiant deed. What is often judged by human standards to be proper or improper in someone else's life is often quite differently viewed from a higher-world standpoint. Admire and emulate the example set by *Challenger*'s gallant crew. What they profoundly executed in one supreme moment clearly categorizes them as heroes and heroines.

It is unfortunate that your governmental structures are interminably unwieldy and resistant to change. The corrupt but tantalizing temptations that human leaders face would take the strength of Zeus to withstand. Although they may have walked innocently into the trappings of government, when they are morally weak their high ideals are soon transformed into cold-hearted, calculating, power-seeking displays. Those who fail to practice self-discipline and highly principled values in accordance with Universal Law soon fall prey to tempting morsels set by the Dark Lords to entrap them.

Unnoticed by the majority, a change is underway. Old workhorses who pull the plow of Earth's harness from an unenlightened stance will soon be replaced with young, vigorous, spiritual idealists and a fresh visionary glow seldom acknowledged outside society's private domains. As the world moves into the dawning days of a golden age, the unpolished, the unspoiled, the unsophisticated, the sweet innocent elements of the human family will assume the rein of power.

It takes a concerted effort to locate people of vision, moral integrity, and courage who are willing to expend their rich spiritual treasures on the draining energies associated with authority in government or megabusiness. However, the mere presence of a spiritually gifted human creates a vortex of positive radiating energy that offsets the disruptive influences emitted by negative individuals. The teacher whose majestic vision, courage, and tenacity culminated in her becoming a *Challenger* astronaut and crew member is an example of the power of a positive-motivator.

Unsung heroes and heroines abound on Earth, yet their names, if noticed at all, are tucked quietly away in human-interest columns or act as fillers for the evening news and are soon forgotten. Unfortunately, the majority tend to sharpen their wits by focusing their attention primarily upon the tawdry events that dominate the media's interests.

In light of the above, it behooves you to contemplate the following: Suppose you were to suddenly float out of your body and find yourself standing before the angelic members of Earth's Spiritual Hierarchy. What would you tell these all-knowing celestial beings when they challenge you to explain the thoughts that motivated your human life?

On Suns and the Nature of God

Energies emitted by extrasolar stars are continuously merging with Sol, Earth's sun. The harmonics of the galaxy in which we all live is predicated upon the ability of the many stars or suns to vibrate in unison. The individual hum or song of the planetary bodies reflects the level of spiritual enhancement of their particular sun's "spiritual personality." The intensity of a sun's attunement to Source or God is identical to the degree it reflects Divine Potential. This remark is best illustrated by, if one may be so bold, visualizing God as a physical body. Initially, the vibrancy of God's omniscient presence illuminates as cosmic dust, foundation material from which stars are created. Omnipresent Cause then structures Divine Light and Sound (vibration) into physical manifestation, planetary bodies, moon bodies, comets, and so forth. Prevalent life—animals and plants—form at the same vibratory light-sound density as the planet or moon upon which they live, which is predicated upon the resonate hum of the system's sun or suns.

As you come to a clear understanding of Love-Light as the basic universal energy component, as foundational material for manifesting stars, you will learn to intuit Earth as a mirror image of the moon, Mars, Europa, Saturn, the sun, and so forth. Matter, regardless of its vibrational rate, has an underlying compulsion to return to Soul Light in an upward spiraling fashion. Spiritual evolution can thus be construed as God evolving God, Perfection evolving Perfection.

Manifest universe is made up of layer upon layer of whirling concentrated zones of purified energy vortices. Specialized regional vortices enable planetary bodies, solar systems, and galaxies to continuously refine their vibrational pitches in agreement with the harmonics of the greater Celestial Song. As cosmic energy ebbs and flows, it reinforces the instinctual urge of matter to refine its internal hum and to strive for absolute essence of Being in perpetuity.

Sol is currently enveloped in an intensified vortex of magnified energy. You may view the obscurity of this remark by considering the power of your inward drive to consummate Self's greater purpose—indeed a Holy quest.

Bypassing no thing, waves of purified cosmic energy spread throughout the universes, capturing all the multi-faceted by-products of Creation, from one-celled organisms to complex solar systems and entire galaxies in their ever-widening nets. Earth is currently caught in the final stages of an energy enhancement, that is, energy squared to energy squared, a high-powered galacticwide wattage system that will eventually culminate in her transformation to a fifth-dimensional light-density planet. Lower-force energies that have kept Earth locked in the cradle of the third-density spatial spectrum are rapidly dissipating. In the transformative year of 1987, Earth began to absorb accelerating amounts of purified stellar energy. Eventually, in one climactic moment, her attention will become riveted upon a vibrational directive issued from the core of the Central Sun. Reaching maximum velocity, her entire physical mass will be propelled into the rapturous interludes of the higher-dimensional planes.

As predicated by Universal Law, all beings are able to adapt or not adapt to evolutionary cosmic events. Those opposed in their heart of hearts to dramatic spiritual change, those who have not prepared themselves to assimilate the refining energies, will be transported with other like-minded individuals to a lower-dimensional planetary system where status quo remains status quo. All beings are free to feed upon deteriorating morsels of negativity until they make a conscious decision to evolve. Minute self-examinations, alterations, and adjustments must be made if one is to complete the ascending journey that culminates in the Light of Celestial Home.

As the harmonic substrates of a given system, galaxy, or universe are modified, a celestial invitation—a specialized summons—is sent to every inhabitant to evolve or not to evolve. You may think that Soul retrieval and relocation on a universal level would be an exceedingly complex undertaking. Nevertheless, it is easily accomplished. To illustrate: You have learned that the material from which the universe is formed is light and sound

(Aum). Humans are in the third octave, where base creative substance gravitates in a natural alignment that is negative-pole attracted or positive-pole attracted. To ascertain the magnitude of individual Soul emissions, Spirit simply initiates a sweeping scan of Love-Light energy available on any given level.

Because of the extreme polarities that exist on Earth, a substantial jolt of Love-Light energy is required to transform human negative-pole thought into positive-pole thought. Transformation is initiated in the heart-mind of an individual who then experiences an escalating desire and intent to formulate greater purpose. "What you plant so shall you reap" is best defined as positive or negative energy actualizing like energy.

Universal Law allows you to be exactly as you choose to be: either a negative-charged spirit or a positive-charged spirit. Neither commitment predisposes you to celestial approval or disapproval. From an evolved viewpoint, negatives and positives are complementary components of That Which Maintains equal part to equal part equilibrium within the dense vibrations of the lower universal substrates.

Creation's Purpose is best described as God-seeking-God, Omniscient Perfection evolving Omniscient Perfection. As microcosmic manifestations of God's magnificent ecstasy, humans are endowed with an underlying urge to discover the perfect portion of Self that radiates omnipresent Love-Light. Those who prefer to indulge in negative forms of cosmic-force energy seek God through reverse-thrust attraction. Though they may initially favor a circuitous route to return to Source Generator, negative-entranced souls eventually realign and merge into the refined Love-Light realms.

Activities deemed sinful or evil by society's standards are a compound of the illusionary bondage that has kept humanity in captivity to the Dark Lords. This situation came about in ancient times when they captured humans, who subsequently began to toy maliciously with the unlimited possibilities inherent in applied cosmic energy. If, at your current state of spiritual development, you could observe the balanced rhythms of the harmonious multilayered universe in action, you would see Love-Light used as the primary building material from which stars, planets, and life are formed.

Because the doubting majority secretly lack conviction that they are capable of attaining Soul evolution and a return to innocence, they are essentially predisposed to composing life's elements from a wide variety of negative thought-producing products. As a result, the powerful energies that fear-drenched humanity emits have polluted the once-pristine air and water of its planetary home. Simultaneously, humans exude an awkward, scattered imbalance of primary positive-to-negative essentials that threaten the stability of the entire solar system.

Humans stand in energy opposition to their own best interests whenever they allow fear's qualities to override their instinctual desire to live good, compassionate, love-filled lives. Essentially, fearing humanity stands in opposition to evolving humanity. As a result, a malady of unquenched spiritual hunger exists planetwide.

Ever-resourceful Creation patiently equalizes all areas of cosmic imbalance. As members of a primary planetary species who persist in sending waves of disruptive energies onto the delicate stellar grids, today's humans are under notice from the Spiritual Hierarchy that they have reached a point of negative saturation.

To many it will appear that the following remark is carelessly outlined, even blasphemously structured. We emphatically state, however, that the darkly evil force that thrives on your immature planet in a quite excellent way serves as an antagonist that causes those who illumine Love-Light on Earth to shine all the brighter.

A call is sent out to humanity from the Regency star council to be about evolving its individual and collective Soul essence. Seek nothing less than the perpetual warmth of Cosmic Hearth.

Seek! Purposefully seek! Urge yourself to radiate as brightly illuminated as a midday sun. Seek Prime Creator with the focused attention of your entire being.

In outlining the original transcript of this essay, I attempted to present complex data as simply as possible through the resources available at the time of Patricia's early awakening. Since then, the sentence structures have been upgraded as appropriate to her developmental growth and understanding.

Malantor, Intergalactic Fleet of the Solar Hum, Arcturian Star Command

Arcturian Star Council transmission: The continuation of this essay on suns is a journey into understanding that cosmic knowledge is being held within the sun's core until the time of humanity's awakening. We will attempt to explain, in an abbreviated fashion, how the various brotherhoods of light and the Office of the Christ are able to store information in a sun or star in a similar way that large quantities of data are placed within a computer for immediate or future retrieval.

Beings of light who have transported themselves across vast distances of space, whose purpose is to awaken you to the full extent of your unlimited potential, are intent upon gathering celestial knowledge and placing it at the disposal of awakening humans. Thus, solar-based essays in this book are as precious as containers of molten gold.

Mental aerobics required to insert telepathic thought into the core of suns are accomplished simply. The mind of one or more beings joined in harmonic concert has the capacity to gather and transmit quantities of thought energies in limitless fashion. Beings of light are naturally proficient in the nuances of telepathy and routinely wrap their minds around exquisite jewels of thought, gather them into brilliant silken packages, and transmit them into space in the form of light and sound.

Like any well-stocked library, various quadrants or sections of the sun contain tomes of specifically categorized information, succinctly catalogued and filed as to type. Although the energies of individual pockets of projected thought render themselves into a multitude of specialized flavors, they simultaneously retain themselves as distinct wholes.

Coordinates of activated solar data are prepared and await enlightened humanity. In the manner that computer documents are transferred from hard drives to disks for permanent storage, information stored within Sol's library is recorded, copied, duplicated, and transmitted to Earth as well as to other planetary bodies within this star system. Historical and spiritual information is stored in pyramids, mountains, rings of stones, wheels appearing in fields, and other sites considered sacred by indigenous peoples.

You who are scholarly are encouraged to formulate mathematical equations on Earth's latitude and longitude grid points, mystical symbolism, and musical notes to establish the manner in which Earth-based artifacts are affixed to solar-grid coordinates. By transposing letters to numbers, you can begin to interpret telepathic communiques. Those who meditate and thoroughly understand that thought creates form have no need of complex formulae, for the doorways of their minds easily access solar-based knowledge. Data stored in the sun's computer core are available through thought to all beings who approach spirituality from a high level of intention. Humans who prefer to function from the tactics of deceit are not permitted access to documents held in sacred trust within the Earth and in Sol's fiery realms.

You may wish to consider this material from a place of mindful meditation.

The Eagles Will Fall from the Skies

Ancient shamanic elders were often endowed with clairvoyant vision. As those prognosticators peered down the corridors of time, they foresaw the coming of an age when a dark cloud of hopeless despair would spread like a cancer over Earth. Weaving their visions into the intricate symbols of tribal mythology, some cautioned their descendants to be wary of a time when ponderous silver eagles would begin to drop like giant boulders from the sky. The accuracy of this prophetic warning is now observable.

Rising into the air like cumbersome and weighty birds, human flying machines propel their ungainly bodies through the sky while their delicate cargo jostles back and forth. The frightening imagery of falling silver eagles is an indicator of an era of quickening time, an epoch of evolutionary intensity.

Since the devastating world conflict of the 1940s, which culminated in a premature rupturing of matter's oneness and the advent of nuclear weapons, men, women, and children of all nations have pleaded with their leaders, their supplicating cries urging "Wage peace, not war!" Yet those who sequester themselves in elaborate marble halls essentially ignore the summons their positions of leadership pledge them to uphold. The tantalizing lure of unlimited power holds sway over all but the most sensible. The hoarse voices and clutching hands of the majority of your government and megabusiness rulers force them into a position of God-evasive silence and spiritual somnolence. Unfortunately, their lack of moral and ethical integrity is not only abusive to themselves but is demeaning to all Earth's citizens.

Humans who hold positions of authority and arrogantly thumb their noses at Universal Law and the practice of unconditional Love as basic to decision-making policy create an enormous energy drain upon Earth's delicate membranes. This is always true when one group wages war instead of peace upon another. The inevitable result of thousands of years of protracted deleterious behavior has played such havoc with Earth's etheric body that an unprecedented accumulation of warped energy threatens the stability of the light grids that connect Earth to other members of her solar family.

Most would be outraged and appalled if they fully understood the ramifications of humanity's unremitting entrancement with the subtle enticements the Dark Lords use to hold humanity captive. Bypassing Love-Light's magnificent potential, the Dark Lords use negative thought forms to encourage a people, already susceptible to fear, to yield to their manipulative, tormenting ways.

Succumbing to the will of the Dark Lords, arrogant, hedonistic humans are destroying Earth's vibrancy for the sole purpose of personal power and monetary gain. Regally strutting about, they are nothing more than unruly adolescents playing a dangerous game. Meanwhile, the emotionally ravaged resemble lemmings determined to plunge headlong over a cliff into a wind-tossed sea. To the ultrasensitive, self-inflicted death beckons as the only means of escape from your planet's terrifying house of horrors.

The propensity humans have for indulging themselves in less-than-delightful activities creates a sense of alarm in more peaceful beings who inhabit the starry quadrants.

To turn to a more positive theme, though you coexist with beings who insist on channeling Creation's radiant energies in negative ways, many of you have tender hearts that pulsate at brilliant light intensity. In spite of the darkness that threatens to engulf them, some of the brightest essences in the galaxy persistently shine from Earth. The spirit bodies of the awakening are like dancing flames. Although it may appear there are only a handful of positive human energy producers, a great many are determined to live in a manner that reflects sublime high Love.

Every year more and more of you are urgently requesting spiritual assistance and psychic protection [see Glossary]. As best we can from a standpoint of noninterference, we grant you these things. Although humans remain essentially unaware of the extent of extrasolar intervention on their behalf, many are becoming cognizant of the subtle guidance that emanates as their inner voice.

Once again, we stress the importance of routine, daily meditation—particularly when confronted with moments of distress and confusion.

A birthing planet vibrating at a lower tone than evolving Earth is preparing itself to receive beings who prefer to embrace greed and power, those who desire to control, possess, and destroy that which is not rightfully theirs. The awaiting planet is far from Earth, but it is not altogether unlike Earth. Humans and other beings who choose to discover God via a backdoor or de-evolution approach soon will find themselves crawling up from the dense sludge of a lower-gravitational vibration. Eventually, these hapless individuals will challenge themselves to dissolve the crusty layers of accumulated negativity that encase their spirit bodies' exquisite lights.

Because the Law of Free Will is delicately balanced by the Law of Cause and Effect, what is sown by the individual must ultimately be reaped. Prior to ascension into the sublime realms, beings who have allowed themselves to slide into the unwary pits of the nether regions must first wholeheartedly commit to recapture and sustain purified light. They must travel up a spiraling ladder that leads to harmonic stabilization. They must precisely adjust the calibrations of their Souls' hum until they resonate like a finely tuned harp.

Because their spirit bodies became entangled in shadowy webs of confusion, it has taken thousands (in some cases millions) of years for implanted starseeds to awaken to the point when they can expend the energy necessary to extricate themselves from the Dark Lords' clutches. One disruptive life after another was more than sufficient to weave a thick karmic cord around their etheric bodies.

To clarify the dilemma Arcturian starseeds face, Patricia's Soul was once a native of the planet Cheuel of the Arcturian star system. During a moment of disdain for Universal Law, she unwittingly participated in an event that culminated in a nuclear catastrophe five million years past in Earth time. Observing from the ports of a starship, she stood aghast as her beloved green home, Cheuel, exploded. Patricia is only one of many starseeds who either volunteered for or were confined to Earth assignment after the horrifying convulsion that destroyed Cheuel.

The horrors of that cataclysmic explosion continue to reverberate throughout the universe. The repercussions of the event resound through the corridors of your subconscious minds and filter into the depths of your sorrow-filled hearts. Cheuel's fiery demise is reflected in your dream images and meditative visions.

Prior to activating her contractual assignment to record telepathic conversations with multidimensional entities, Patricia fervently challenged herself to valiantly protect Earth's endangered plants and animals in thought, word, and deed. Trudging with pictures of her beloved wolves, she talked and pleaded on their behalf. After much contemplation and inner dialogue with her spiritual advisors, Patricia eventually concluded that her path to enlightenment required her to incorporate practices of ego-surrender in order to actively serve Universal Will.

You may think Patricia's behavior irrational. "Not at all!" we reply. If you closely observe the difficult things she has forced herself to do, you will understand that the courage and will it takes for her to grow and manifest her heart's desires are equally applicable to you.

In September 1987, Patricia was summoned before the Regency star council upon *Marigold–City of Lights*, where she came face-to-face with the resonating presence of Earth's Spiritual Hierarchy and the Christ Essence. It was requested that she instill within her manuscript words of hope and Love to encourage you, her readers, to abstain, as best you might, from weaving any further threads of disharmonic thought into the delicate tapestry of your Souls' exquisite quilt. Since that evening, Patricia has endeavored to fulfill her pledge. She suggests you view her as a reflection of yourselves. She is hopeful that her work will inspire you to courageously commit yourselves to serve Earth and her multiformed citizens in a manner best suited to your creative talents and hearts' calling. We echo her sentiments exactly.

We sometimes refer to you who are awakening to the Memories and your starry origins as wanderers. Many of you are somewhat aware you are being called to play an important role in Earth's evolutionary process. Many who have answered their personal summons are concluding that what is true for others is equally true for them. As brief visual glimpses of humanity's multidimensional, universal connections slip through, their hunger to realize all the minute details of their Souls' journeys accelerates. Their dreams and visions are replete with subtle symbolic hints that they were seeded upon Earth from the stars as surely as the pyramids stand in Egypt. As their pre-encoded Memories reactivate, they are manifesting an overwhelming urge to significantly serve Earth.

A mightier baton was never waved than the one orchestrating the awakening. Long have the seeded wanderers dormantly resided on Earth. As they germinate and unfold in full bloom, their inner ears discern the opening stanzas of a great star symphony.

Those who maintain positions of authority in the workings of nations would do well to come to the clear understanding that many "mediocre" people are of multi-star origin. In current Earth time, starseeds are fulfilling a higher vocation than traditional society asks of them. Multigalactic in origin, they are stretching forth to embrace the dynamics of their forgotten Soul Memories. Their numbers increase daily.

The key to activating your internal solar hum is to seek harmonic spiritual balance. It takes but one beat of your heart and one unfaltering footstep to turn in the direction of Universal Light. It is a weary individual indeed who consciously and with willful intent turns away from the golden path after discovering it.

Unfortunately, we find it necessary to document many harsh reminders through many channels before the seeds of human Soul reacquisition can germinate within the heart-minds of the spiritually lethargic. It is a sad commentary on your times that many are disinterested in spiritual matters because they do not want to face collective humanity's critically urgent challenges. Therefore, the record we play will continue spinning round and round as we essentially reproduce one repetitive song.

I, Malantor of Arcturus, came to Earth at the request of the Arcturian council of elders. It is my "assignment" (loose descriptive phrase) to prepare certain documents that are the rightful possession of all beings. My fellow travelers, the entities, the personnel on the thousands of starships in Earth residence, hail from many stars, many galaxies, and several universes. Humans who interact with us as telepathic receptor-senders, such as Patricia, directly cocreate with one or more beings of light whose vibrations are essentially the same as theirs: same note, different octave. Those whose essence qualities match Patricia's include, but are not limited to, Palpae of Arcturus, galactic emissary to Earth, and myself, Malantor, in the capacity of advisory counselor.

The resonant descriptive names of beings in service to the intergalactic fleet shine like brightly lit suns. Their rhythmic tones are incorporated in many magnificent works of visionary art. Ships from the stars have ridden upon the energy waves that glide around Earth since the time of galactic seeding. As parents true, we are ever-mindful of the welfare of our sleeping children.

Cheuel, the Green Planet of Arcturus

Malantor transmits thought via the fluid media of transbeing telepathy. Because mind energy is capable of being recorded, at times we store thought in solar "computer" disks placed in strategic locations on Earth for this purpose. When transmitting via solar disk, we notify Patricia that incoming information awaits by sending her a buzzing sound. Her task is to find time in her busy schedule to tap into the solar-disk data and reconstruct it upon her computer monitor in logic-linear English graphics.

Sweet are the moments allotted to Malantor and Patricia to interact directly, as we are doing in this moment's energy. As I communicate with her, my light-body is floating serenely through the comfortable corridors of *Marigold–City of Lights*. Magnificent is *Marigold*, like a garden bursting with a rich array of unfolding flowers. Her massive hallways are alive with ripe plains of blooming sedge.

An ancient being herself, Patricia-Manitu was a resident of the Arcturian system long before she came to Earth.

Although her Memories of the Arcturian planetary system are almost completely faded, whenever she experiences pain and sorrow her mind easily conjures up horrifying visions of the catastrophe that destroyed her beloved Cheuel. Like many who are awakening to their ties to Arcturus, Patricia's heart-wrenching Memories of Cheuel's final moments are actively triggered by imprints carried in her body's cellular membranes. Picturing Cheuel as debris circling around the Arcturian sun, she erupts in tears as her heart-mind agonizes over the frail state of Cheuel's sister planet, Earth.

The sickening agony that Arcturian starseeds experience when they rewitness Cheuel's death throes lies like weights upon their Soul Memories. Many of Cheuel's ancient inhabitants were Soul-transferred to Earth five million Earth-years ago. Earth school affords these individuals multiple life opportunities to evolve and transcend the galactic-level karma they incurred with Cheuel's abrupt, violent demise. Waves of energies associated with the uniquely third-dimensional Law of Repetition (reincarnation) are a particular gift that Earth willingly took upon herself when she was formed into planetary material for her enhancement to light-body status.

When life's burdens become especially difficult, it is not unusual for transplanted Arcturian starseeds to subconsciously access cellular Memories where their imprints of Cheuel are stored. In times of heightened visual or emotional intensity, they often catch a fleeting vision of Cheuel's untimely death.

For millions of Earth-years, fractured, splintered, dormant Cheuelian fragments revolved around the Arcturian sun. Some of our technological breakthroughs have given our intergalactic "construction crews" the means to marshall the energy necessary to reconstruct Cheuel's remains and remold them in original form. By a simple technique that captures and blends subatomic light particles together, we have restored Cheuel's majestic body to cohesive stability. We entwine and reentwine planetary fragments at a subatomic level by splicing coils of laserlike lights around similar coiled lights.

Located in the Boötes constellation, Arcturus shines like a beacon in Earth's night sky. Her sparkling image is encouraging humans to become consciously aware that it is time for them to assume their places as functioning members of the greater galactic community. Verdant Cheuel is ready for the return of her transplanted children. She has retaken her place as a sweetly humming Arcturian light-body planet, and her vibrant emerald-green essence circles serenely around giant, rosy-red Arcturus.

As an awakening starseed, you are urged to focus your awareness upon the goal to achieve ascension to light-body status by willingly adapting your energies to the practice of unconditional Love as primary in all you think, say, and do. Your inwardly expressed commitment to Soul evolution makes it possible for extraterrestrial solar scientist-engineers to beam uplifting electromagnetic impulses through your body's neurocellular system—an important detail in the awakening process. After your etheric solar batteries are charged, your light-body matrix will activate by itself.

The lingering horror of Cheuel abruptly exploding because of her inhabitants' actions continues to exert a sobering influence upon the entire galaxy. As twentieth-century time draws to a close and a new millennium begins, the accelerating tragedies upon Earth mirror the events that climaxed in Cheuel's explosive death. The Souls of Cheuel's ancient citizenry mutually shouldered cosmic obligations. However, as awakening Arcturian starseeds passionately dedicate their lives to promoting healing of their adopted planet, Earth, the karmic cords that virtually chained them to the past are rapidly dissipating.

I am in ecstasy, for I am one who has been chosen to bear witness to the transcendent moment when Cheuel's long-displaced children return home.

Starship pods in Earth residence proliferate. A vast array of extraworld beings are gathering around Earth's sun to participate in dynamics associated with the vibrational evolution of this entire solar system. Emissaries from a multitude of star systems, galaxies, and universes have formed a cooperative amalgamation whose combined talents are dedicated to assisting Earth's inhabitants in the mechanics of celestial transformation. For the most part, blissfully unaware of the proximity of extraterrestrial starships, the surging mass of undisciplined energy that collective humanity continues to exude indicates to us that the majority remain entranced with a variety of self-indulgent, mindless occupations common to Soul-hungry people. Humanity's ongoing fascination with sad, emotionally unfulfilled, and violent songs, stories, and movies is a reflection of its neglect to incorporate applied spirituality as the main thrust of its social, political, and religious institutions.

A Brief Note on Astral Travel

Many of you are able to achieve a conscious point of physical, emotional, and mental relaxation and, at will, profoundly slacken your physical bodies' tight hold, intentionally thrusting your astral bodies free. Adepts at astral travel can purposefully activate a time envelope when, if only momentarily, they can escape from the deluge of disruptive vibrations that are the predominant feature of humanity's cacophonous society. Those who learn to release their light-bodies to float as free as eagles must first execute a form of self-hypnotic suggestion. As they tease their brains into trancelike states, they gently coerce their logical minds to surrender the hold their physical bodies have upon their spirit bodies.

An initial voyage into the gravity-free astral planes may evoke a variety of intense emotions. Novice travelers often experience an uncomfortable sensation of being suddenly and unceremoniously liberated from their bodies. Those who are not yet proficient in mastering the techniques and mechanics of astral travel often experience impressions upon their emotional bodies that are less than uplifting. Indeed, the experience can be quite strange and very terrifying. The limited experiential sense range of the physical host is not immediately amenable to separating itself from the cellular components of the body's layers. The exact method of relinquishment is not always available to the cognizant mind, and an out-of-body experience may seem to occur outside the mind's control. For the unprepared, it is not a comfortable sensation to abruptly detach from the known confines of the physical body.

Although the ability for astral travel is a natural phenomenon, spirit release is not properly understood within the limitations and prejudices of human religious traditions and current science. Because an out-of-body happening may occur without any impending warning, the psyche of the uninitiated in the art of astral projection will be unprepared to experience physical body disconnection. When one is unceremoniously propelled free from the cagelike environment that holds a protein-based body in material form, the sensation of sudden freedom is incredulous and startling. Nevertheless, the time nears when transforming humans will become acutely aware that they are spiritual substance encased in physical substance.

The longing within to become as a cheetah flying free upon legs that gobble up miles in a second is a natural human urge. The hearts of those who are infirm or broken in body, confined to a hospital bed or a chair with wheels, have an even greater yearning for physical freedom. Although humans have a tendency to cling tenaciously to their bodies, the truth is the majority feel imprisoned within them. To overcome this dualistic polarity, an important task facing those who aspire to spiritual ascension is to achieve emotional and intellectual acceptance that the true nature of Self is as a spark of brilliant, eternal Light.

Psychedelic and Medicinal Plants

Early in the development of Earth's vegetative cover, plant species with different healing properties were brought by extraterrestrial intelligences to provide budding humanity with easily obtained curative agents. It is particularly unfortunate that in today's world, greedy, spiritually immature people are short-sightedly usurping the natural healing properties of mind-altering plants for monetary gain. Many are beginning to view nature's greatest gifts as a means to momentarily enhance, deaden, or otherwise escape the physical, mental, and emotional pain that permeates "civilized" society.

Indigenous people meticulously selected psychically endowed children to serve rigorous apprenticeships under the guidance of highly skilled elders, guardians of the tribes' sacred knowledge. Before assuming the obligations and privileges of full-fledged shamans, however, they were thoroughly schooled in the attributes of psychedelic plants and medicinal herbs and were taught to concoct them into potions for healing and for use in sacred ceremonies.

Now the responsibility all humans share for maintaining the natural world in harmonic balance has been delegated to a handful of dedicated individuals who maintain a somewhat rudimentary knowledge of plants as originally intended. In today's world, potent plants traditionally reserved for sustaining the health and well-being of entire communities are being used by the self-indulgent as a means to momentarily escape lonely, fear-filled lives. Humans who routinely abuse the psychedelic properties of medicinal plants are placed in the precarious position of perpetuating karmic obligation in future lives. Those who habitually misuse drugs eventually fall prey to diabolical beings who inhabit the shadowy astral regions. Improper ingestion of highly potent plant substances escalates mental confusion and emotional turmoil within the psyches of long-term addicts. Perpetual abuse of the body temple that was designed by God as a perfect receptacle for the Soul's journey creates a degenerative situation within the body that culminates in disease, insanity, and eventual death.

Your physical form and genetic heritage were adopted by your higher Self as appropriate vehicles for modifying and harmonizing cause and effect and to provide situations to enhance Soul evolution. Most enter life with their exquisite Soul-knowledge virtually intact. However, their delicate neonate minds are immediately assaulted by saberlike thrusts of negativity erupting from the general population's fear-driven minds. The electrical synapses that connect their newborn brains to their superconscious brains are soon slashed like weeds before a sickle.

As you dream through this experience called "life," your purpose is to fulfill the terms of a contract you entered into with your higher Self before birth to remove the sticky influences of the past and to attempt an override of accumulated energies that encase your spirit or auric body. If your resolve is to move into the future karmically unencumbered, you will best achieve spiritual clarification through a loving attitude and a sincere attempt to live a good life.

In the complex, strained events associated with Earth's leaving her third-dimensional moorings and moving into the domains of light, it is imperative that you, too, release desires and expectations limited to third-dimensional reality. The times call for an acceleration in personal healing. To help you prepare for light-body ascension, we recommend choices that promote health and emotional well-being through the appropriate use of psychedelic drugs and medicinal herbs. A critical, thorough study of literature available on the ancient uses of medicinal herbs and aromatherapy is recommended for those who are drawn to alternative healing arts.

Evolving Earth, Evolving Humanity

I, Malantor, am a fifth- and sixth-dimensional light-energy being visiting Earth from the Arcturian solar system. My purpose in contacting Patricia is to create a human format through which I might introduce myself. We are mutually inspired to bring your spirit an elegant uplifting. Our purpose is to implant a block of ecstatic hope so firmly within you that you may easily access it as solid, life-foundation building material.

Although the significance of galactically inspired writings is not easily accessed by the logic-loving mind, their more profound qualities are easily absorbed by the intuitive mind, or heart-mind. The deeper meanings of the essays may or may not assemble before your eyes in a smooth, flowing manner. Their cadences may toss and turn in your head in a syncopated rhythm. You may find yourself valiantly struggling to assimilate subtle cosmic information not altogether in line with humanity's scientific and religious teachings. Whatever means you use to integrate these data, understand they contain harmonic by-products carefully designed to resonate beneficially with your diverse personalities and perceptions of metaphysical knowledge.

Elevate all fear-based residuals that linger within to a higher plane. Learn to ascertain short-term and long-term ramifications of thought and their subsequent actions, for the concentration of fatalistic pessimism that emanates from the planet's surface is so negative that, from our view, it appears as a solid band of dark clouds wrapped tightly around Earth's entire circumference.

One purpose for contacting you is to inspire you to clarify dire predictions in a positive manner. Maintain a higher perspective when anxiety and despair threaten your peace of mind. The big picture is that Earth's picturesque skies are strung with radiantly flowered multisystem starships inhabited by God-oriented beings who patiently await an invitation to assist you. You will not access us, however, through the use of radios, computers, or televisions. To contact beings of light you must finely hone your intuitive minds' telepathic abilities.

Unfortunately, global leaders remain resistant to change and are demonstrably unwilling to serve and uplift their people through standards of behavior in accordance with Universal Law. As they attempt to maintain a stranglehold on the status quo, they fail to conduct themselves in harmonic agreement with Universal Mind. Generally, human interchange reflects prime-level Oneness only at times of high-wattage energy such as during holy-day celebrations, weddings, births, sudden tragedies, loss, and death. Sadly, as the initial surge of powerful energy dissipates, human capacity to indefinitely sustain an attitude of compassionate unconditional Love subsides sharply. At their current level of cosmic maturity, humans as a whole are totally unprepared to cooperate as a united world family. The results are an escalating increase in crime, plague-like illnesses, and generalized decay tormenting inner cities. Befuddled by a stagnant bureaucracy itself immobilized by public inertia, disinterest, and spiritual ignorance, the masses are unable to cope with the severity and extent of their problems. As the megacity environments smolder like kegs of dynamite attached to short fuses, the inevitable outcome should be easy to predict by even the least astute observer.

It is time for humans to buckle down and merge their divided nations into one mighty, love-based cooperative. The only avenue remaining to avert worldwide environmental, technological, and economic disaster is for humans to actively practice the simple tenets of Universal Law.

Earth has been slated by the Regency star council for vibrational evolution. Her gross physical substance is being manipulated and maneuvered into position to assume her rightful status as a light-resonating planet. She has begun settling her maturing neonate body into a canal of impending birth. In a very real sense, as she is born into regions of refined space, she will return to her celestial family in a state of childlike innocence.

As Earth's light expands, she will transcend her karma. She will no longer carry the burden of providing sanctuary for war-loving, spiritually ill-at-ease souls. As her vibratory mood purifies, every pore of her rocky body will radiate particles of light. Her water will run clear; her air will sparkle and dance; her land will hum with the delicate notes of a thousand strumming harps. As she attains the tranquil levels of the fifth and sixth harmonics, her light brilliance will increase tenfold. Because of her advancing luminous radiance, Souls wishing to claim Earth as their planetary home must maintain themselves at her vibratory level.

As Earth moves through stages of vibratory retuning, you may periodically catch a glimpse of rainbow-hued shimmering. You may shudder involuntarily, as if a ghostly apparition had just fluttered by. If you turn quickly, hoping to get a clear glance of the illusive specter, your optical sensorium may feel strangely stimulated, as if your visual clarity were blurred from peering into the depths of a warped mirror. As unexpectedly as it appears, however, the strange phantom fades. You may not realize that you have touched upon the rim of Earth's transformative body, the point of impulse where she rapturously absorbs light. If your heart-mind accepts the reliability of your experience, you may find yourself straining to capture another glimpse of the dancing rainbow image your peripheral glance was privileged to enjoy.

In the next years, you will find your hesitation to strive for spiritual enlightenment much sweeter when you contemplate the enormous effort it took you to attain it. As you move into the higher-reality realms, you will learn to discern the tricky cords of energy that weave in and out of Earth time, linking past time to present time and present time to future time. Eventually you will comprehend the illusionary nature of third-dimensional linear time. You will also learn to identify the sublime multihued cords that link Earth and the planets of this solar system to the sun and the cords of light that link the sun to the stars.

When time is expressed as past-present-future, the natural rhythmic tones of the spatial cords are constantly threatened by disruptive, abrasive sounds the inattentive collective emits. Humanity's chronic problems with agitated instability have deposited layers of tarnished thought residue upon the light matrixes of Earth's less-resilient grids. Because enormous spatial strain is associated with planetary realignment, it is vital for humans to participate in maintaining Earth's oscillating structures in harmonic integrity. In preparation for Earth's impending dimensional transfer, her corded grids are carefully monitored and polished by galactic maintenance crews who keep themselves busy repairing her damaged ethereal substrates.

Rigid-thinking people are severely limited spiritually and seemingly prefer a binding of roughly woven tradition to the silky robes of enlightenment. In humans, there is a generalized stubbornness to move beyond the safety of fear's known qualities. Because of their hesitancy to practice the demands of unconditional Love, humans lost the ability to move freely among the stars. Long ago they withdrew into themselves. Loss of paradise, as described in Judeo-Christian sacred texts, is symbolic of the ramifications of your ancestors' ancient decision to sever ties with their greater galactic family.

Humans are a distrustful species. Their prevalent attitude is to mold themselves into a variety of institutions and nations whose leaders' prime concern is to claim rightful dominion over the lives of others. In ancient times, humans lost the ability to actualize when they succumbed to the insidious energies of the Dark Lords and essentially broke off all effective communication with beings of peace and light who inhabit the subtle worlds.

After thousands of years of accumulating deleterious karmic energies, humans could no longer consciously co-create their world through principles of Divine Manifestation. As a consequence, most prominent thinkers became stuck on the rather quaint notion that authentic reality is made up of compacted physical matter. Those who profess to believe in the reality of spiritual worlds are often looked upon as delusional. This skewed perception of the universe has become so deeply embedded in the human psyche that most religious and scientific traditionalists are like stone cast in cement—rock solid and virtually immovable.

Humans have manipulated and twisted the simple tenets of Universal Law into a complex system of self-indulgent, short-sighted rules and regulations, a strange set of formulae that primarily benefits the few. The cumulative result has cost the collective dearly, as is reflected in the chaos that represents the accepted norm. Historical and religious tomes gathering dust on the back shelves of libraries detail the consequences of centuries of warring, tyrannical behavior.

Though these times appear to be inauspicious, the final chapter of human history is yet to be written. You may still resolve your oppressive difficulties through cooperative, inspired effort. In truth, all your environmental and social problems would instantaneously and peacefully resolve if you were to come together as a body of One and emit one massive surge of compassionate Love. Yes, in one brief second God's Holy Kingdom would establish itself on Earth. Until then, because of humanity's generalized spiritual inertia, the Federation for Planetary Affairs, Intergalactic Brotherhood of Light, will continue to maintain active coordinates for Earth's dimensional transfer as directed by the star councils and Spiritual Hierarchy for this spatial quadrant.

As you seek us out, be it only one, two, or three, you grant us privilege to quietly and gently contact you. Do not, however, presume to hand over your responsibility to commit to fulfilling your life's specified purpose, for to assist you in any other fashion is not our duty. Our role is only to act as guiding elements that aid in the development and maturation of your spiritual growth. Therefore, it may not seem immediately apparent that the stressors which bind you to third-dimensional reality are easing. Our agreement is to help you prepare for light-body ascension. If you intensely desire to participate in personal and planetary healing, your passion to initiate transformation will set the energy to do so in motion.

We clearly convey that there is an urgent need to restore the fractured plates of the world's ailing continents to prime health. All fragments of Earth's sorrow must be disintegrated and its bits and pieces washed clean before she and her resident children can rise into the radiant arms of perpetual rapture. Although we maintain active vigilance over her, for the most part we remain hidden from view.

It is our privilege to promote a greater understanding of Universal Law on Earth. We want you to know that the mood of despair permeating the human community is not an emotion common to those who will populate Earth's future.

Creation Is a Multidimensional Experience

Shallow bogs and deep caverns are abodes for creatures from which "civilized" society chooses to disassociate itself. Retreating for safety's sake from the communities of their larger biped cousins, wee "fantasy" folk long ago drifted into the fading mists of alternative time, taking many precious facets of primordial wisdom with them.

Intellectuals consider mystical environs and tiny creatures as preposterous stories told to stimulate children's vivid imaginations. As the centuries wore on, science- and technology-loving adults became more and more unimaginative. As they lost the ability to conceive of alternative realities, they began to claim once-pristine Earth as their sole and rightful territory. As a result, unusually formed beings were driven farther and farther away from humanity's sterile environs.

Truly a frightened species, humans have closed themselves off from any substantial interaction they might have had with a multitude of diverse beings who inhabit the invisible worlds around them. To protect themselves from unknown reality, they erected a barricade of contempt around their self-centered empire. Sadly, as the impenetrable walls of self-imposed exile thickened around them and their living space became increasingly cramped, only a few adventurous souls dared step over the narrow causeway that separates humanity from the vast lands of a greater reality.

As humans' peripheral vision narrowed and they were no longer able to perceive anything beyond third-dimensional space-time, they began to focus attention exclusively upon their own busyness. Virtually unaware that translucent beings occupy living space exterior and interior to their own limited reality, most humans lost the ability to directly communicate with "fantasy" people.

It is vital for all beings that humans lay to rest the oddly egocentric belief that they occupy Creator's central attention. It is time for humans to commit as much energy to merging in sacred Oneness as they do to separating themselves from themselves.

Source Creator manifests Itself in every life droplet, every tiny wiggling shape, every star, every planet, every asteroid that moves through the heavens. Every living thing carries within itself the seeds of potential Eden. Creator gives abundant sustenance to all the diverse beings that inhabit the great star nations. Each embodies principles of Divine Love. Each is part of a greater whole. And, although being One, each remains wonderfully unique.

Upon the tapestried backdrop of never-ending space, Celestial Artist eternally paints. Seek Its name; Its name is unnameable, unfathomable, but may be spoken in phrases of sound and color incorporated in Light-Love Intelligence. Seek to honor and respect all creatures, for enlightened beings regard all life forms as Star Maker's children. It serves no purpose to envision oneself as being of greater or lesser import than another.

No matter the density of its vibratory ring, eventually every being crawls diligently, if somewhat slowly, back to Central Sun, Cosmic Home from whence Soul originated. Even those who become entranced with Creation's balancing side, the planes of darkness, will eventually turn tail and earnestly scamper back to sacred light.

All life is precious. Life is Creation's greatest miracle, no matter what form it takes. To expand your capacity to appreciate life's myriad forms, we suggest you take a few moments to inwardly contemplate upon beings of light who dwell upon starships. Then pause and consider the wee people, those miniature beings who peer at your gigantic bodies from the safety of their secret lairs.

Fifth- and sixth-dimensional light-entities, extraterrestrial inhabitants of starships in residence Earth-base, resemble pinpoints of multihued lights. Though we play freely among the magnificent star fields, in reality we are not that different from you. As I communicate with my sister Patricia, I am lying in blissful repose upon the spinning golden orb of brilliant, flower-laden *Marigold–City of Lights*.

Adonai this day's beauty.

Let Not the Light Dim

There springs hope within the breasts of mystics and dreamers that, eventually, all will be well. Hope's refined resonations stir within the hearts of those who awaken. Courage, as an outcropping of hope's exquisite energies, stretches its vibrant tendrils to wrap the gentle in nature in its supportive vines.

We urge you to face life in an unflinching manner, even though the future may appear vague and uncertain. Though the tones of negativity's lowered notes seem to be escalating, we tell you that in only a few years the predominant energy swirling around Earth will reflect only Love's ecstatic colors. Earth Mother is assuming a state of divine grace. To facilitate her transfer into the light realms, pods of starships are kept busy pouring rays of "computerized" colored lights onto and into Earth's body to heal, stabilize, and refine the vibrational matrix of her energy grids.

You who are challenging yourselves to assume an active role in species and planet acceleration are rapidly evolving. Self-motivated, spiritually focused individuals whose primary intent is clearly defined to serve Spirit are supplied with the means to activate their auric bodies. They naturally radiate Love-Light's pure essence. Often unbeknownst to themselves, delightful humans who completely immerse themselves in their passion to know God intimately begin working in harmony with beings of light. These humans' subtle anatomies, or chakra systems, capture and anchor streams of sweetly scented, softly colored lights that constantly ply around Earth's surface. Using their chakras as light-wattage filtering systems, they dispense light downward and outward in gentle waves to penetrate Earth's restless bulk with beams of healing energy.

Mass consciousness is heavy with anticipation. The natural environment is in imminent danger of collapse. Because of the nature of mind (thought directs energy), empathic individuals are particularly prone to these rays of negativity that bombard Earth's communication airways. Unwary but psychically energized individuals are particularly susceptible to periods of despondency, chronic emotional instability, and phases of acute, debilitating fear.

Hypersensitive individuals must learn to intuit that those with deteriorating values are transmitting primitive, garbled waves of telepathic thought into the planetary airs. Although it is impossible for even the most astute to maintain a constant state of heightened awareness within the confines of third-dimensional linear time, we caution vigilance against any influence that attempts to weaken the brilliance of your light pulsations. Dark entities are determined to match your mood to their oppressive temperaments. They constantly inject pulses of poisonous negativity into the unsettled mass body. As a result, the planetary air reeks with the putrid odors of undisciplined, destructive, hate-charged thoughts.

Despite the building gloom, we encourage renewal of personal optimism. Hark to the sweet, melodious songs of each new day. Indulge in the protective dress of your childhood's innocence. Freely and introspectively immerse yourself in nature's delightful garments. Be of good cheer. The times are rich, exciting, and bursting with spiritual opportunities. Oh, precious gift, you were born to be a part of them.

Go then into the streets and summon those you meet to listen for the majestic song the starships sing. Rejoice in the loving presence of your galactic family. In the face of adversity, bravely persevere in mirroring hope's fine features. Accept your role in these wondrous times, that of sky warrior, eagle of the new dawn. You who are attracted to this material are a starseed, a light-Souled being from the stars. It is your purpose to plant seeds that will eventually germinate as the foundation for a magnificent new society. History's strings are being pulled, its final threads drawing to a close. Earth Mother is preparing herself for an uplift in octaval hum.

Hold high the precious energies of hope in these despairing times. When your tender heart flutters with pain and suffering, do not allow the light to diminish. That seemingly small point of light within you, your insignificant-appearing Self, is an important beacon for the starships. The untapped power of potentiality that resides within you is a mighty sword forged in God's fiery furnace.

Starseeds, we know how impatient you are for dramatic events to occur. You are pushing us to perform, you who are so anxious to transform, ascend, and become One with us. We realize how difficult it is for you to stay constantly tuned to our subtle telepathic resonations. We are aware of how life's distractions place you in a turmoil of dreary details that often block your expanding abilities to sense Spirit's presence. We know for which you yearn. Your hearts are open books to beings of perpetual light.

Meditate and will yourselves to a higher vibration. Eagerly dwell upon what you understand as Divine Truth. Allow your minds to soar unencumbered. May the magnificent mass of twinkling stars called Milky Way remind you of candles flickering at a sacred ceremony, a ceremony in your honor. You, the children of the stars, are the focus of our delight. You have only forgotten that you are an integral link in a vast, unbroken cosmic chain. You are essential threads in the golden tapestry Star Maker weaves.

Imagine you are visiting Malantor of red-hued Arcturus. We are taking a contented ride upon a humming, rainbow-hued starship. You are satiating yourself in the arms of Divine Ecstasy. What bliss!

Teleportation and the Power of Thought

Teleportation—the movement of physical mass from one location to another via adaptations inherent in the power of thought—is not prohibitively difficult. As humanity's will allows, the simple feat of transporting people and objects from place to place via the energies of thought will be a normal occurrence. Although the ability to instantaneously translocate is generally looked upon as a form of trickery used by magicians, the common use of teleportation was never meant to be limited to the adept at sleight of hand. Essentially, it is no more complicated to spontaneously relocate than it is to focus a beam of concentrated thought from your mind to a distant point. Unfortunately, humans are so infatuated with metallurgic-plastic motorized technology that their boats, planes, trains, and automobiles have relegated them to traveling in dangerous, slow, and awkwardly maneuvered vehicles. Conversely, fifth- and sixth-dimensional beings of light stationed around Earth are quartered in palatial, environmentally viable, planetlike starships.

The interiors of our starships are ripe with life. They are sweetly textured with rich landscapes that vibrate in harmonic agreement with many suns and many planets. Majestic, crystalline, floral-essenced, and atmospherically perfect, our multilayered starships are planetary monitoring stations, healing stations, and gathering arenas for all activities associated with our diverse natures.

Not unlike sailors stationed at exotic ports, we have maintained Earth residence since life's inception upon your planet. Our primary ship, *Marigold–City of Lights*, is but one of many starships in residence Earthside. Enormous, *Marigold* is a true miniaturized planet. Geographically, we have berthed her in recent times above the vast energy swirls that are continuously rising from the northern portions of the Western hemisphere.

In a display of ecstatic Oneness, our collective minds spontaneously reposition our ships at mutually agreed upon points along the stargrids. Or, free of the encumbering shells of our space vehicles, we are capable of instantaneously transporting our light-bodies through space. Unfettered as the wind, we freely glide upon the shimmering stargrids. We resemble bright, bobbing musical notes as we dance our merry space dance along the humming interstellar cords.

A certain expenditure of energy is required to achieve instantaneous teleportation. There is always depletion whenever power is used. Usually, only a moment's layover after a long haul is needed to reenergize a starship's crystalline hum, much as you revitalize your bodies with nutrients and sleep after a particularly lengthy excursion.

Although we are primarily concerned with Earth healing and transformation modalities, we remain constantly attentive to the thoughts of our starseeded human associates, many of whom have conscious recollection of a personal link to Arcturus. Nevertheless, the slow process of arousing from the long sleep of repetitive life cycles finds many starseeds in a state of confusion. They struggle to access their starry Memories and their latent psychic potential.

We have come to harvest our crops, to gather the precious starseeds who have completed their current-life Earth assignments and to transport them to their home stars. Those committed to ascension in this lifetime will eventually achieve higher-dimensional realms as their light-bodies emerge from their physical bodies like butterflies exiting cocoons.

Most of Patricia's family of friends were birthed upon Earth many aeons ago, yet their hearts sway and dance to the rhythmic vibrations of planets and suns their minds vaguely remember. Soul Memories of those who are Arcturian-connected resound sorrowfully with echoes of exploding Cheuel. Periodically, haunting images of their regal home star and its many planets imprint upon their inward visions. Though they are now in Earth bodies, their vibrational frequencies hum in rapturous tones with the magnificent sonata of rosy Arcturus.

As do all suns, Arcturus resonates in complementary pitch with the Soul patterns of her planetary children. Some Arcturian planets are as verdant and green as Earth is, with creatures whose essences are similar to but much lighter than Earth creatures. Some planets, by human standards, would seem barren and devoid of life. To Arcturians, however, their rocky contours are a delight of sweetly scented gases and brilliant splashes of colors that lift and swirl in the planetary winds.

The Blue Crystal Planet is our dominant planet. That is, her celestial song embodies harmonic components characteristic of all our sun's satellites. Raw solar energies swirling planetward from the depths of the giant Arcturian sun are captured by light-absorbing crystals on the Blue Crystal Planet. Massive crystals raise their pointed heads so high they seem to touch the rim of rosy-hued Arcturus. Strategically placed, these obelisk-shaped energy-storage crystals are kept steadily humming. The delicate but highly charged emissions of the crystal towers serve the Blue Crystal Planet's inhabitants as primary power generators. Within the crystals' depths the planetary hums are born—delightful, ethereal songs that make life possible within a light-evolved star system. Never depleted, never wasted, energies held within the crystal giants remain uniformly stable. As they waft their sweet colors, scents, and hums externally, they immediately shift and regroup internally. Crystalline-powered fuel is the energy source for all technologically advanced planetary systems: Arcturus, Pleiades, Sirius, Antares, Andromeda, and so forth.

Because of Arcturus's celestial location, Blue Crystal Planet serves the Lords of Light and the Intergalactic Brotherhood as a principal gathering arena, a midway point where members of the star councils discuss and implement interstellar business matters.

Equal in scope to the beautiful crystals of Arcturus are the magnificent crystalline fields of the Pleiades. Like giant radio antennae, enormous energy-refining crystals connect via light the Pleiades with Earth's sun system. The Pleiadian crystals capture critically disruptive energies that constantly stream into space from Earth's inhabitants. With a great inhaling cosmic breath, these crystals draw unsettled thought emissions inward, where they are cleansed of potentially dangerous particles. Then, with the crystals equally vigorous exhalation, purified thought energies are returned to Earth.

Beings from planetary systems that use crystalline energy as primary power are particularly sensitive to thought's destructive elements. Among the citizens of this galaxy, Earth's humans are considered an especially thought-excitable species. For the most part, humans are unaware that their brains resemble super-amperage batteries. It would not occur to them to consider the ramifications of undisciplined thought. Spinning skyward, their discordant thoughts attach like glue to the delicate stellar cords. Thoughts' images slide up and down the grids like electricity traversing a copper wire. They whirl this way and that like billions of erratic gyroscopes. Left unattended, these projectiles would snake along the stellar grids until they rained upon the innocent inhabitants of other solar systems. The Spiritual Hierarchy closely observes all negative-positive fluctuations arising from Earth and instantaneously directs the intergalactic crews to diffuse the impact of prickly thought upon less agitated beings.

Humanity has traditionally aligned itself with fear's noisy thoughts; it primarily projects assault-level sound. Fortunately, these negative-charged reverberations are somewhat counterbalanced by the sweet passion of positive, love-charged vibratos. If this were not so, long ago the intensity of unbridled thought would have ripped open the fragile fabric of Earth's crust, and humanity's elegant planet mother would have torn asunder in a hideous crashing maelstrom—Humpty-Dumpty effect. Spun like balls hit by a bat, the Soul bodies of Earth's slumbering inhabitants would have flung outward upon the delicate spatial highways. With nothing to hinder the speed of their momentum, they would have traveled through space like bullets. But permanent disintegration of energy is not possible under Divine Law. Eventually, the bits of microcosmic light representative of Earth's unfortunate Souls would have settled upon a planetary ball better suited to the growth of cosmically immature essences.

Communities of the New Millennium

Groups of like-minded people will gather in pods as the energies of the new dawn settle into place. Many of you are already finding yourselves drawn to live in small, self-contained, self-sustaining communities during the transitional years. As Earth Mother moves into the harmonic realms of the higher fourth dimension, your favored styles of living will be quite different from those common to third-dimensional life. As you become cosmically enlightened, you will be through with the deprivations of agitated loneliness, the result of doctrines preaching that humans are separate from God and from one another as well. As you free yourselves from the ravishes of false judgment, jealousy, and pernicious desire, all your self-other interactions will be based on peace and unconditional Love. When you reach peak ability to profoundly perceive the Christ Essence in perpetuity, you will bond as one glorious family of living light.

New-millennium communities will establish mission statements on principles of mutual trust and compassionate consideration. Friends and neighbors will joyously communicate in an honest, open, forthright manner telepathically. As one-to-one mind-thought is openly embraced, all misunderstanding and interpersonal misconceptions will cease to be and the haunted memories of such things will fade into the recesses of the past.

As the new millennium progresses, you will fail to find it enticing or pleasing to confine your bodies in energy-stagnant, box-shaped buildings and transportation devices. Resource-efficient technology will provide unlimited power, which will allow you ample time and the means to reflect upon and express the full potential of your uniqueness as a divine being and citizen of an expansive universe.

Boring, demeaning, discouraging chores that dissipate your vital energy will give way to cooperative endeavors among many acting as One. Each moment will be precious beyond measure, every appealing second a treasure chest of unlimited possibilities and soul opportunities. When meeting, you will hail one another from a position of mindful alertness and nurturing self-other esteem. As the energies of the new millennium become firmly established, an enlightened Earth citizenry will consciously interact as family with other inhabitants of the great star nation.

As Earth moves out of the dense vibrations of the third-dimensional regions, your bodies' cellular makeup will increasingly lighten. Gravity's chains, like shackles that have kept you karmically tied to your planet, will fall away. Dis-at-easement will be nothing more than a vague memory of a tortured past. Your bodies will no longer be subject to age, decay, fatigue, blotches, stains, or other disfigurements that plague your lives.

New-dawn people will resemble buzzing, productive, peaceful, contented bees. Work will be a leisure, and leisure a blessing. Resplendent as if she had donned a lush, freshly laundered gown, Earth Mother's every aspect will be vibrantly beautiful. She will be covered with magnificent flowers and all kinds of fruits and vegetables. Your homes will be tranquil residences, snug and elegantly attired. No longer will you be held in bondage to "make the payment." You will be freed from the backbreaking need to produce and consume a seemingly unending supply of commodities necessary for survival. As you learn to instantly manifest all you desire from the cosmic ethers, you will become secure in the knowledge that you live in an abundant and loving universe. But we caution: clearly thought-indicate what you truly want, for the universe is expansive and extremely accommodating. All things sought are eventually granted.

We who reside upon magnificent cloudships are quite aware that an almost overwhelming supply of manufactured goods has, since the onset of the Industrial Age, accomplished little more than place greater hardships upon the people. Sadly, those who do manage to attain monetary security are as haplessly held in bondage by the trappings of their opulent lives as are the desperately poor. Few wealthy individuals escape the illusive trap that their affluence grants them of preferential status and social privileges.

Earth Mother will soon render complete her karmic debt. As she gracefully winds her way through the depths of the cosmic ocean, she is being maneuvered into the peaceful intonations of a higher-dimensional octave. Eventually she will cease producing sustenance for those who insist on living outside the Law of Perpetual Harmony. In the greening years of the new dawn, by necessity all who inhabit Earth will preferentially embrace precepts of Love-Light in everything they think and do.

Are you one who understands the concepts of cooperative, creative endeavor? Are you eager to live a spiritual life in perpetual bliss with other radiant inhabitants of the great star community? Are you committed to establishing peace as an Earth constant? If so, you are among those who, one fine day, will discover yourselves propped upon the grassy knolls of a serenely transformed planet. You are among the magnificent ones, for you know life is meant to be grandly lived and that ecstasy is meant to be a normal state of being, not something sporadically experienced.

It is virtually impossible to communicate every detail of the radical shifts occurring in every aspect of society. During the years of the changing, cling tightly to hope, faith, and trust as if you were holding a tangible object, for their powerful energies will serve to comfort and sustain you in the manner of a favorite stuffed bear during childhood's stormy times.

Childhood. Carefree days when your small-in-stature self dreamed an easy dream of the new dawn's poignant promise. That innocent aspect of Self once swayed to the delicious rhythms of your Soul's sweet song. Set free the wee one that lives within you! Let it spin, whirl, and dance! It is slated to accompany Earth as she loses herself in rapturous abandon, the gliding rhythms of a galaxywide celestial promenade.

Did you cast aside your innocent self's delicious visions of a wonder-filled future as your "maturing" ego deposited itself into the frame of a large-boned adult? Are all your youthful dreams tucked away because of the seeming impossibility of manifesting them?

Passionately protected as any beloved babes, in the new-dawn era you will experience love as a constant, not as a sometime thing. Love's soft whispers will cease tearing at the delicate fibers of your hearts. Your sorrow will dissipate as the recesses of your broken hearts are filled with the ecstasy of childlike laughter. You will know peace. Your tears will be only for an outpouring of abundant thanksgiving. You will cavort under the ocean's surface with dolphins and whales. You will sail upon the thermal winds with eagles and hawks.

Pledge your star brothers to you. That which is written will come to be.

As Droplets of Water Are Humans

Commencing life as falling drops of rain, precipitation is birthed in the form of beads of water. As a raindrop spatters upon the ground, it may find itself settling upon the rocky contours of a high mountain peak, nestling around the roots of a tree or bush, or caressing a delicate-hued flower petal. As the droplet begins exploring its new environment, it notices the presence of other droplets. Soon the tiny raindrop and its newly discovered companions begin to blend as one into a wee trickling riverlet. Seeking companionship with others of their kind, many riverlets merge to form a clear mountain stream. Gurgling in delight, they swirl and dance as they flow into a shaded pond to which forest creatures come to drink. After a rest in the eddies of the pool, the droplets begin to tumble and whirl as they are pulled into the slopes of a steep canyon. Tossing and turning along the roughness of the river bottom, the droplets' long journey eventually brings them to the channel of a riverbed. After many days' travel along this watery course, the droplets attain their final destination as they converge into the mighty substance of an ocean.

When a droplet molds itself into the contours of a great ocean, its purpose is fulfilled. A microcosm of water blended as One with the many realizes its destiny, for the nature of water is to seek water's source. Though integrated in the ocean's immensity, the integrity of the individual drop is sustained.

Humans resemble drops of rain. They are like flakes of snow. Remaining unique unto themselves, their individual characteristics are, nevertheless, vital to sustain the energy of the overall human collective.

Malantor's primary purpose for bringing forth the rather obtuse symbology of this essay is to inspire you to seek Creator Source as diligently as droplets of rain seek the sea. Time is short for humans to harmonize their multiplicity of national, racial, religious, political, and social groups into one harmonious, world-encompassing unit, a task that must be accomplished before the luscious fruits of cosmic citizenship may be digested. You must surrender your historic preference for separatist behavior. To assume your rightful roles as citizens of a great galactic federation, you must first make peace among yourselves, for those who prefer the ravages of war will not find themselves traveling with beings who have attained the stars.

These are accelerated times. Those who cling tenaciously to rigid, outmoded beliefs are so narrowly focused that they are unable to see beyond the cramped confines of the third dimension. Certainly, they are incapable of comprehending that the stars and planets teem with life or that the universe is densely populated with intelligent, peace-loving beings. Be prepared: The truth is much stranger than any fictional narrative, more wonderful than any mystic dares to dream.

We remain confident, for even as the outline of this transmission takes form upon the computer screen, many humans are simultaneously awakening to the fact that Love-Light is universal foundational energy upon which telepathic communication with extrasolar beings of light is established.

Earth Stewards

Taunt not other creatures! With your expanded awareness, understand the extraordinary role that each animal and plant plays in nature's exquisite drama. Reconsider the belief that humans were granted privileged status over all things. Be it clearly understood: Your primary function is that of chief planetary steward. All Earth beings, not only animals and plants but rocky substances as well, are dependent upon you to diligently love, cherish, and nurture them as do all wise, responsible parents their offspring.

As the new millennium shifts into gear, the planet body will enter a phase of extended grace. As humans perfect their innate ability to communicate with one another telepathically, they will also experience the unfettered thoughts of other life forms. How delightful, how exquisite, how fulfilling!

Long ago, in an effort to halt all honest thought exchange among Earth's diverse inhabitants, the Dark

Lords erected an energy barricade that effectively ended all inter- and intraspecies mind communication. Now, your brain's capacity to absorb and transmit information is growing because daily you feed it so much more information than did earlier generations. Truly, you are an evolving species. Rigidly held scientific beliefs are giving way to a broader concept of Earth's interdependent biosphere, and the advent of quantum physics is stimulating many scientific investigators to explore the universe as a dynamic, multidimensional organism.

When Earth's fourth-dimensional transfer is complete and as humanity ripens cosmically, extinct animals and plants will be given an option to genetically reintegrate into Earth's refined energies. Humanity will have an opportunity to petition the Regency star council for the return of individual animals and plants. A courtlike atmosphere will prevail. Issues pertinent to universal harmony will be contemplated gravely. In contrast to youthful humanity's naive attempts to control nature, a cosmically mature people will revel in life's exquisiteness. Humans will represent themselves in one integrated voice. They will agree to regard, honor, and respect all living things. Reverently and softly, the melodies of unconditional Love will drift into the heavens.

Cosmic citizens who conduct themselves through the use of Love-Light's energies do not require monitoring or crisis intervention. As humans awaken to their place as members of the great celestial community, they will practice compassionate love toward all creatures. As humanity achieves spiritual maturity, starfleets will come and go reciprocally, for when humans majestically blend in uni-versal (one-song) harmony with their galactic family, they will have unlimited access to the grid system that connects the stars. Together we will glide from constellation to constellation, from galaxy to galaxy, from universe to universe—delightful adventures not for just the rich but equally affordable for all.

The tones of our transmissions may appear harsh to a people driven to maintain structural conformity, those who are solely occupied with the necessities of shelter, food, clothing, and back-and-forth transportation. The by-products of your material-based society have presented you with many serious problems requiring urgent attention. Nevertheless, our aim is to encourage, not discourage. As such, we have nestled nurturing overtones of hope within these documents.

Know this: Beings who live by the precepts of Light-Love harmonize in perpetual unity. We share universal abundance equally, for what is available to one is equally available to all. A light-evolved being never attempts to control the will of another. Star-council delegates mutually agree to serve as One. We do not perceive ourselves as rulers or heads of state. We do not envision ourselves as privileged. We are coordinators and facilitators of functions to which we specifically resonate, that is, the vibrational patterns adaptable to our Souls' purposes.

Spiritually attuned citizens of the greater galactic community have equal voice in all cosmic "business matters." Every opinion, every thought is deemed equal. At fifth-degree cognitive level, communication is telepathic; nevertheless, the sanctity of the individual is never violated by those who live in blissful union with Omniscient Mind. "Things" (that which may be likened to inanimate objects) may be had by all, altered, expanded, or diminished as individual will predicates while concurrently fulfilling the Will of the Greater One.

Eventually, a solidified, unified Earth citizenry will evolve from out of the dust of your crumbling economic, government, religious, and military structures. Aeons of organizational inadequacy are beginning to melt away like icebergs floating in a tropical sea. The horrors of thousands of years of undisciplined living are tumbling from the sheer impossibility of sustaining their unmanageable weight. Human society is stressed to maximum sustainability; it heaves and strains. Many calamitous events have begun, triggering those who slumber into a frenzied attempt to pin together the deteriorating shroud of their dissolving illusions.

In our efforts to awaken you to the gravity of your situation, which, in fact, has become obvious to even the least observant, we warn you that the misappropriation of habitat and vital functions of plants and animals is very serious. Your responsibility as emerging galactic citizens is to hold all creatures with the tenderest of care, love, honor, and respect. First, you must remodel a world long fascinated with the ravages of war into a garden of perpetual peace. What, blessed ones, would you think if extraterrestrial beings were to treat you as you treat one another? Would you not deem us vile and evil?

Assuredly, your most important task is to love one another unconditionally. Unconditional Love is a medium of stellar energy. Unconditional Love reflects starlight off moons and planets. Starlight is a reflection of Supreme Intelligence, whose dissemination of unconditional Love plants seeds of light and life throughout the many universes.

On Birthdays

It is commonplace to experience a wide range of emotions and activities associated with self-other birthday celebrations. However, in the new-dawn times, the pleasurable practice of treating one's incarnating "birth" date with almost holy-day ritual will end. Nevertheless, it remains a fine thing, on birthday occasions, to spend a few quiet moments contemplating one's rich genetic heritage and pondering humanity's ancient connection to the stars—meditative exercise most beneficial in helping you unlock the vast treasure trove of Soul Memories secreted within your subconscious mind.

Blessed ones, in a tranquil mood allow your visionary eye to focus upon images of the past as they arise before you. Make a conscious effort to clarify and identify the pictures and to assimilate the knowledge that accompanies them. Meditative concentration techniques are important tools for developing the abilities of your computerlike brain to access and store higher-level information.

The design of this essay is to startle you into accepting yourself as much more than a one-life being. We urge you to take a giant step toward acknowledging yourself as Soul, as ultimate Being.

As the light-bodies of Earth's diverse inhabitants became entangled in the gravity-producing karma associated with the fluctuating energies of Earth's third-dimensional position, they began to cling perilously to physical life. Because of the grievous difficulties they bring upon themselves, the Christ Essence has always surrounded the Souls who incarnate here with sweet radiances of pulsating light. Like Earth and her parent sun, you, too, are tenderly clasped in the warm embrace of a magnificent stargrid. A crisscrossing, ethereal bridge of flower-scented, humming light securely anchors the star-suns and their attendant planets in the arms of perpetual grace; luminous Light-Love emanations perpetually surge forth from universal Sun-Soul Central.

At some point in Soul's evolutionary journey, your I Amness or higher Self became attracted to the magnetic negative-positive polarities that are indicative of Earth's gravitational situation on the solar grid. As your Soul-Self became entranced with Earth's rich diversity and unique multidimensional substratums, your light-body settled down to explore itself by means of repetitive sentient beings. As a result, your Soul Memories became trapped in a maelstrom of life-death hysteria as your spirit became bound in the dramas that attend fear-based third-dimensional beings.

Although it may appear that we have gone off course on the topic of birthday celebrations, we reiterate: Our primary purpose is not to congratulate you for your tenacity to attain a certain age in life but to broaden your experiential expression of Self as Soul having a human experience.

To provide yourself with some measure of intelligent guidance through life, before entering a physical body your spirit set up certain specifics for date of birth, time, location, name, and family. These particulars are carefully incorporated into the cellular matrix of the prebirth fetus. Your astrology and numerology charts are excellent resources for helping you comprehend and clarify these data. Most humans, however, continue to hold tenaciously to the conviction that there is only one life to be lived and that past, present, and future are made up of a series of separate yet somewhat related events. A curtain of illusion spreads around their light-bodies. These unfortunate beings have adopted a vaguely identified form of emotional and mental balance to convince themselves that they are safe and sane. Few consider themselves magnificent beings composed of particles of radiant light.

To achieve a clearer understanding of Self as Soul, envision yourself as a being formed of light, an ethereal being who has decided to undertake a long, arduous journey. Entranced with Earth's beauty, you halt to investigate its exquisite pleasures. Too late you realize the inhabitants of this beautiful planet are quite dangerous and cosmically backward. Seeking shelter in the growing darkness, you find protective lodging in—what appears to your newly arrived senses—a medieval inn. You quickly discover that the muck and gore of disease, grief, and death are commonplace. You are horrified by the brutality, the brawling, and the cursing of the people. You search for some means of escape. Too late! You have forgotten the whereabouts of your crystal traveling pod. Even more alarming, your lightness of spirit body has become trapped in a dense physical form. Exhausted from the effort to free yourself from the heavy gravitation pull of this world, you eventually succumb to the relative safety of drifting cosmic somnolence.

Caught in the process typical of life on third-dimensional planets, you move in and out of one life form after another. Each new birth triggers drowsiness, a chronic form of Soul Memory amnesia. Your neonate self struggles for a great deal more than life's first breath. As your wee baby bottom is roundly patted by those in attendance at this auspicious event, the first sounds issuing from your lungs is a scream, a gasping gulp of panic as, once again, you find yourself sinking into a mire of spiritual sleep. All that you understood as a light-body being takes flight as the Memories are sucked out of your baby brain like air escaping from a punctured balloon. Much of the tears of a newborn is from the pain of feeling itself slip into the subdued form of a third-dimensional body—like caging a wild, free spirit behind the bars of a dungeon.

Interestingly, from life to life the date of your birth becomes a marker for important festivities. Death, the marker that sets you free, is the cause of anguish and sorrow in those left behind.

In spite of these difficulties, third-dimensional physical life is wondrously advantageous to Soul. Every life experienced on a material-based planet affords Soul an opportunity to refine, rebalance, and upgrade its light resolution.

Continuing your meditation, envision Earth as a cosmic schoolhouse. You are a freshly scrubbed child, apple in hand. Eagerly, you take your seat. You sense rising excitement, for you know you have come to gather wisdom in preparation for returning to the stars. Clear your desk. Make ready for the appearance of a very special teacher. Now a somewhat austere but loving entity enters the room. This awesome individual is looking directly at you. Hesitantly, you challenge yourself to rise. You face your teacher with confidence. In a voice ringing loud and true, you clearly recite your cosmic lessons.

The portrayal of teacher before student, and student, in turn, before teacher, is a symbolic reflection of the higher light-form's ability to interact with the physical form—Self communicating with self. Paralleling the imagery of Self mirroring self, the stars and their accompanying planets image one another, for as a sun illuminates its planets, planets return light to their sun.

Reflections and Images

Focusing on your intuitive eye, visualize a time when you unexpectedly found yourself standing before an unflawed mirror. The reflected image may have momentarily seemed that of a stranger, yet there was a feeling of familiarity. It can be disquieting to abruptly come upon your duplicate without time to settle into the posture normally assumed when intentionally gazing into a mirror.

Although it is slightly upsetting to see one's naked face, it is even more disturbing to observe oneself as a twin of the Planet Mother's polluted countenance. Uncomfortable with her unhealthy reflection, Mother Earth has begun a process to remove the scabs of industrial pollution that cover her careworn face. She is readying herself to slough off the disease and decay that torment her delicate skin. Although humans skitter from here to there in a vain attempt to perpetuate their illusions, the unsubstantial images they have erected are dissolving like phantom reflections.

It should be evident to even the least astute that the synapses of Earth's nervous system are being altered and that her vibrational harmonics hum a progressively refined melody. She is extremely volatile, yet the intense nature of her vibratos are so magnificent that she will eventually entice even the most reluctant ear with her captivating song. Those who survive the upcoming deluge are destined to take a grandstand seat at her greatest performance. Many of the awakening would clearly prefer to bypass the opening stanzas of her prelude, preferring to move right into the rich symphonic arias, for they know that as a Wagnerian opera is built upon chord structures that crash like lightning and thunder, the passionate stanzas that mark the beginning notes of this concert will echo into space with almost violent intensity.

Before the final curtain, you will have an opportunity to assist in orchestrating the colorful score. You will write a few rapturous notes. You will conscientiously insert the light of your arousing energies into the core of Earth's being. Your intention will define the rhythmic tones of her symphonic masterpiece. The greatest production ever performed is underway, and you are its principal producer and director. You will pluck the strings of its harmonics. You are composer, conductor, musician.

You cannot bypass the promise of the future by turning your back upon its reflection. You can no more escape the forward times than you can avoid imaging yourself when gazing into the quiet waters of a forest pool.

When humans begin visualizing themselves as Mother Earth sees them, the imagery of their self-protective posturing will crack. The tottering foundation they have built their structures upon will shatter and fall. Humans are perched like a mass of tightrope contortionists high above a crowded tent where the ringmaster is announcing the main attraction. Prepare yourselves! The full attention of the universes is fixed upon you. Center and balance yourselves upon the rope. Run a preliminary check of your safety nets, for the strength of steel will not protect those who fall backward in the face of unmanageable fear.

For assistance during these auspicious times, consistently keep in telepathic contact with your personal light-bodied counselors. Call them to you, for they await your summons. Your spirit guides are misty beings that stroll like soft shadows beside you throughout the turmoil of your days. They appear as physical substance in the chambers of your dreams. Their gifts of advice are precious beyond measure. Do not deposit them in some never-looked-upon place, for their teachings are preparing you to return to the stars.

As you read the opening chapters of this manuscript, you learned that a long time ago I, Malantor of Arcturus, struggled with the restrictive contours of many incarnations. You were told that I rose from the muck of a sodden sea to ensconce myself in a multidimensional light-body. My evolutionary song may serve as a reflection, for one day you, too, will ascend to the stars.

As you prepare yourself, routinely take time in the busyness of your days to breathe in, to absorb tinctured essences of exquisite love and joyous laughter. Anoint your body with these substances. Allow your spiritual vitality to bud forth and bloom. Open the portals of your hearts in trusting anticipation that a glorious new-dawn sun is nestled on the horizon. Hark to the soft voice of the majestic being that dwells within you, that yearns to be free. Lift your thoughts high above Earth's limited perceptions. Send greetings to the clouded starships and absorb the rays of loving light they reflect. Carefully scan the night sky and note the pulsing red, white, green, and blue lights that reflect the images of starships parked before the lights of distant suns.

We come not to mock you but to embrace you with a large dose of hope and to assure you that peace is to come to your planet. Our ships hover above you. We announce our presence in clouded form as the sun ascends. Cozily we tuck the white clouds around us as we dock our starships in their interiors. Periodically, we may slip through a spatial portal and sail through the sky like bolts of flashing multicolored lights.

Don't strain your eyes trying to see a green bug-eyed monster. We who ride the space chariots are formed of beams of radiant light. Our minds shift and turn and leap around the stars. Our light-bodies dance and slide along the pathways that weave through space—those humming, scented grids of magnificent light. We may swaddle ourselves like protected babes within our crystalline ships, or we may float unencumbered, as free as a seed carried upon a summer's breeze.

We attempt to communicate with you in such a way that our words will reflect the unconditional Love we have for you. We want you to become fully cognizant of our presence. We are real! We are not just shadowy forms that taunt your dreamy imaginations. We are more than costumed figures that leap from the pages of books and science-fiction movies. Be aware: Many of the wispy clouds floating through the sky are berthing pods for multidimensional starships.

As I transmit my thoughts on reflections and images, my sight-unseen light-body has entered the living space of my Soul-sister Patricia. The silent song I sing is delivered next to her outer ear. Though the delicate fibers of her mind's telepathic resonances can pick me up from far-distant Arcturus, her emotional being is feeling warmly embraced because I am so physically close. She is endowed with awe, for to have her etheric companion in the room next to her gives her a sense of overwhelming comfort.

The Age of Revelation

Although many perceive the results of contemporary political and religious dissension as being excessively evil, this has long been foretold not only in holy Christian scriptures but also in many other sacred texts. These are the dawning years of an age of energy transformation. Prime orchestrator of this revolutionary era is the Christ Essence, who, for the most part, resides in His light-body upon our starship, *Marigold–City of Lights.*

Marigold is an ideal perch for observing the doings of Earth's most heartbroken, most belligerent beings—humans. In many guises the Christ Essence effectively honors the diverse needs of all people. Often, He assumes a bodied form to bestow primary teachings, blessings, and encouragement to the discouraged, afflicted, and hopeless. In a very real sense, however, He has always been here. His Essence has always resided in your hearts and minds. Only those who suffer from spiritual stupor, those who deem themselves separate, will be startled by His coming.

Although a series of catastrophic-appearing occurrences are scheduled prior to the cessation of this phase of human history, humanity's greatest fear—that of total annihilation—is not a planned event. For example, if any nation attempts to unleash full-scale nuclear war upon its neighbors, the entire intergalactic starfleet will appear and the Christ Essence, in a voice resonating thunder and lightning, will broadcast the dictates of Universal Law for all to hear. He will state that Prime Directive allows no room for any group to disregard the integrity of Universal Law. Nor does the Law of Free Endeavor find the masses agreeing to self-destruction by the manipulations of a few power-crazed individuals. Thus, the abrupt appearance of extraterrestrial spaceships would not overstep the free will of the majority.

Nevertheless, a limited number of nuclear events may yet take place. Earth's beautiful skies over several major cities may fill with burning ash and raging fire. Ancient seers, those with the ability to traverse down time's corridors, clearly observed these things. They also saw an invigorated Earth, abundantly strewn with prairies, with splendid fields upon which a gentle lamb peacefully nestles with the subdued form of a magnificent lion. They correctly intuited the new-dawn world: The image of the Lamb was that of Christ Come Home; the lion, humanity's savage nature transformed.

We urge you to a deeper appreciation of Universal Law. We urge you to understand that the metamorphosis taking place within Earth's physical substance—her transformation to light—is not self-limited. She accompanies all planetary bodies and their moons within this solar system, even the sun. This galaxy, even into the far regions of the universe, is refining vibrationally. We all are moving closer to That Which Summons. Like a great clanging bell, the Milky Way is being maneuvered into position to execute a massive resonation shift.

Telepathic relay hails from the cloud tunes of the red sun. The recordings of Malantor of Arcturus are not necessarily original; indeed not, they are duplicated in many documents throughout the ages. These writings are basic universal-flow energy. We who observe you resemble droplets of light. Inexorably we travel; our journey is complete when, in unison, we enter the Sea of Eternal Light, the core of Central Sun, where all Souls eventually blend with the captivating radiance of Omnipotent Source Light.

I still this vibrational note to contemplate, in my own manner, the anticipated rapture of that supreme moment.

Fear Us Not

We know how your stomachs become queasy, how your muscles and nerves become taut, whenever you seriously contemplate the possibility of beings flying around Earth in shiny silver saucers. Unsettling images are imprisoned in the minds of a curious species who take enormous delight in frightening themselves. Visions are replicated in a multitude of horror, high-adventure motion-picture and television productions. Indeed, it is strange that humans, who are so hungry to love and be loved, focus so much of their attention on negative-emotion entertainment.

We observe your passionate subconscious longing for the return of your ancestors from the stars. Yet most of you remain virtually unaware of how close contact is. Stand with outstretched arms before the sky in a field that has no trees to hide behind. Openly greet us. Have no fear! Exude excitement and joyous anticipation! We are no farther away than are the fluffy clouds.

It would comfort and reassure you if you would take time to study the ancient legends, traditions, and pictographic artifacts of indigenous peoples. If you correctly intuit them, you will discover they are steeped in symbology of our primordial presence. Your heightened awareness will give you pause to wonder why simpler folk took for granted what modern sophisticates dare not acknowledge.

Do you fear the return of a beloved family member when you are physically separated for one reason or another? To embrace a similar attitude toward your family from the stars would greatly expand the parameters of our anticipated meeting. Gravely, we reiterate: You-we-I are One. All beings are created from the same master plan by the same Master Architect. All of us have been gifted with forms best suited to the environmental integrity of our planetary homes. Our life designs are all manifestations of Soul essence; thus are we shaped in God's image. Soul is Soul, no matter how or where it takes form—and you would be surprised how many forms there are. Although all facets of being are individuals, they remain component aspects of Omnipresent Unity.

We encourage you to understand that telepathic relays between Malantor of Arcturus and Patricia of Earth reflect our perceptions of an expanded reality. Remember, too, that Malantor once was human. That which is Self well recalls myriad fearful things that grasped at my bowels and brought vomit to my Roman warrior's lips. Now Malantor is privileged to represent the Arcturians at galactic star-council functions. Once I became light-body intact,

I remembered how I swung from one frightened life to another until death's illusion brought an end to my difficulties. After I left fear's un-love-ly substance behind, I quickly advanced to my present state of energy enhancement. This being, Malantor, who caused blood and gore to flow from his human family as he arrogantly marched with Caesar's legions, now rides in ecstasy upon a multidimensional starship.

Those of you who glory in the "artful" accouterments of war are cautioned to acquaint yourselves with Karmic Law! Energies associated with acts of aggravated assault caused my Soul much pain and spiritual disharmony until I began to realign my light-energies. Insolence held me in bondage, and a narrow focus of attention brought me inordinate sorrow and suffering.

The telepathic writings of this session are energized by the Arcturian sun. It is Malantor's pleasure to be among those who resonate with Patricia. Others who resonate at her frequency include Palpae, Special Arcturian Envoy to Earth; Tashaba, a Sirian cat-energy; and Quantra of Arcturus, a solar scientist. You may not be able to fathom how many minds residing in many places can communicate as One Mind. Nevertheless, putting purified energy into an open and receptive mind is easily accomplished by beings of light.

We are eager to share our knowledge with you. It is not our desire to leave you with unanswered questions. Even if our manner of speaking seems curious, we urge you to study the manner in which the words lie upon the paper. As you learn to understand underlying energy you will begin to notice how the Language of the Sun transforms into an English writing style that is unique to Patricia.

Malantor-Patricia mind connection concludes this essay. We are One, the starship riders and our human family. We are One.

Adonai.

The Nature of Families and Relationships

Moving outward from the warmth of their birthing sun, newly hatched Souls gather around forming planets to construct a light-bridge among stars. From the womb of Soul Genesis the seekers are born, Souls destined to wander from world to world along the galactic corridors. Swirling along webbed strands of gossamer light, Soul casts itself into the spatial ethers. Swept up in the humming tides of oceanic space, neonate Souls set sail in all directions.

Begin to fathom individual Souls as Oneness-in-Being, parallel energies that connect all things to Source Creator. Strive to heed the summons of Omniscient Soul. Become alert to the presence of That Which Is One within you. Become aware of the proximity of those whose presence evokes positive or negative emotions. Observe how a "chance" encounter with a "stranger" will often elicit a sense of familiarity. Etch these images upon the maps of your mind. These beings are your "like ones." Entities—both human and otherwise—who resonate within your emotions and cause your latent Memories to stir are your Soulmates, your traveling companions through time and space.

As your Soul-Self lowered its vibrations into third-plane physical manifestation to don the cloak of an embodied humanoid, you laid aside Memory recall of those to whom your Soul is most intimately tied. Why? Because, when you first came to Earth, you agreed to place the Memories in limbo for many lifetimes. Although you always incarnate with some of your Soulmates (many remain in the spiritual realms of the astral plane; others exist in even higher dimensions), you do not consciously remember your magnificent Soul relationship with them. Now the foggy mists that have covered your Memories for many, many generations are beginning to dissipate. As your vibrations refine in conjunction with Earth's movement into the fourth dimension, you will begin to remember.

Open yourself to greet all who "chance" to cross your path. Those who grace your days and nights are your higher Self's dearest companions to the "beginning and ending" of "time."

As your eyes alight upon a familiar face, whether it be family, friend, or stranger, welcome any small flicker of response, even though tangible recognition seems to hover just outside the realm of clarity. Though your cognitive mind may not grasp what is before you, awareness is constantly coming down from your Soul in the form of symbols. Stay alert! Memories can be triggered by something as minute as the way another wears his or her hair, the way the eyes look, or the way a voice sounds.

To set those intuitive sparks flaming, give validity to seeming odd moments of synchronicity. When coming upon others spontaneously, it is likely you have "stumbled" upon a member of your I Am Self, a being you have danced with lifetime after lifetime for millennia—indeed, since Soul conception.

Doped with the drug of spiritual slumber, your mind was covered with a curtain of forgetting. You simply do not remember how closely interwoven your spirit body is with that of others. Religious doctrine has embraced separatism so thoroughly and for so long that most humans fail to comprehend the nature of Soul relationship—that they are beings of light melded in eternal Oneness with God's Essence.

Frustrations and endearments, a mixture of deep pain and sorrow interspersed with moments of supreme joy, characterize most of your relationships. Earth's majestic yet tattered garment mirrors the fluctuating qualities of self-other interaction, for the unbalanced thoughts and wavering emotions that disturb your harmony and peace are quickly absorbed into her energy-sensitive body.

Relationships are of paramount importance to humans. Now, many practical resources are available to help you establish loving, harmonious self-other associations. A desirable goal is to encourage yourself to aim for unconditional Love at all times for all sentient life, not just for humans. Practitioners of the spiritual arts must strive for a high level of interspecies-extraspecies relationships. Acquire the ability to focus, express, and receive unconditional Love. Those who embrace this elegant, evolved mode of living dwell in a state of contented rapture—essential Oneness.

With the same ease that your physical body senses the world around it, beings of light experience their environment as undulating waves of purified energy. With this in mind, as your intuitive intellect begins to honor the highly spiritual aspects of energy, you will find yourself whistling a brighter tune as to the nature of greater reality.

Although human leaders have been aware for many years of the warnings of Earth's extraterrestrial visitors, they persist in planting undisciplined pockets of unstable energies—such as nuclear waste, environmental pollution, and negative thought forms—into Earth's geologic strata. Eventually, these pent-up primitive energies will reach magnitude force that, if left to themselves, would seriously damage the integrity of the continental plates. One of our purposes in directly contacting you is to caution you: The predominant thought forms that are the basis of your unenlightened relationships must be raised to a higher caliber. Those who fail to do so will not accompany Earth when her grid connectors link with the upward-spiraling vibrations of the celestial hum.

Although we prefer to telepath information that centers around your rich, powerful, creative potential, we must also address the unfortunate poverty of being that so often dominates your relationships: the perpetuation of the illusion that you are only marginally connected to others. Caught in the torments of chronic Soul Memory loss and suffering from the pangs of paralyzed psychic inertia, you live in a world of pervasive loneliness. Suspicious thoughts, pride, frustration, anger, jealousy, and judgment have taken root in Earth's lovely garden. Nevertheless, the gentle ways of love endure. In spite of the oppression that, at times, seems to overwhelm you, love's tender fingers remain firmly wrapped around your hearts. You are recognized as being among the galaxy's most ardent lovers. Your innate capacity to use love's energies periodically opens your hearts' hidden contours. Then you are like eagles spreading their wings before the wind. As you fervently display love's energies, brilliant light radiates from your heart chakras and circles Earth Mother in its powerful, healing, warm embrace.

For a moment, set aside your heavy burdens and float upon the wings of rejuvenating, loving thought. Allow your mind to relax. Deliberately bring wispy images of love's magical ways before your inner eye. Image yourself in a serene landscape, a mystical place where fairies dance on drops of drifting moonlight, where bobbing fronds bend to touch tranquil waters. All that disturbs the stillness is the soft sound of a wee snail gliding over the bottom of a stream. Give your churning mind permission to unwind, to rest within this tranquil setting.

I, Malantor, languish in a state of peaceful contemplation upon the planetlike starship *Marigold–City of Lights*. In a state of ecstatic joy I stroll through *Marigold*'s flowered, rainbow-hued corridors. You who dwell under Earth's billowy cloud-filled skies are not dissimilar to beings of light who seek to emulate Source Creator from the confines of extraterrestrial starships. Soul urgency to blend with That Which Compels Light is a universal constant. We all seek Oneness with God, supreme Soul integration. We have long struggled to become as you find us. We, too, have lived multiple lives upon untold planets lit by the fiery light of billions of stars. We did not obtain Oneness of Being and light-body ascension without an arduous climb through the energy dimensions. What is true for us is equally true for you. We would have you understand that you are a vibrational reflection of essence beings who preceded you into the magnificent worlds of light.

The magnitude of this Memory imprint is to stir you to awaken to your long relationship with the entities of your galactic family. The foundations of our mutual Oneness, the broad aspects of our timeless familial relationship, are fibers of vibrant light from which our Souls were originally woven.

Adonai for this day's dream.

To Touch Spirit

Any day that puts spiritual matters on the back burner of importance is a grievous day. Deluded by high-tech society, humans are becoming increasingly distracted from acknowledging spiritual practice as life's most dynamic function. Although it is not unusual for humans to tap into the light realms when praying, the main focus of their prayers is often aimed at personal gratification rather than at commitment to enhancing Soul's higher good. Rarely do individuals living in industry-based societies consider themselves spiritual devotees, and those who do are considered suspect by the general population. Fewer still have the slightest comprehension of the extent of extraterrestrial influence on humanity's temporal affairs.

Malnourishment of spirit shrivels your heart cords. Emotional and mental chaos has become a common denominator in the world's richest societies. Perpetuating the generalized level of chronic frustration is an unbalanced attraction to physical rituals—sexual contact, jogging, swimming, climbing, sports in general. Overindulgence in work, play, relationships, food, alcohol, or drugs squeezes out any remaining moments for meditative clarity on the nature of Soul. Wherein, then, lies life's splendor?

Your spirit body derives nourishment from contemplating Light-Love and from absorbing Earth's beauty. Spirit's nature is a driving passion to unfold the heart center, to allow an opening to experience life as a magical gift. Physical, mental, and emotional endeavors are meant to complement spiritual activities—not take their place.

Humans have a tendency to deplete their energy on physical survival and fleeting pleasures. Soul's predominant desire, however, is to ripen and mature its light vibration. Although it is fine to appreciate and surround oneself with the good things in life, to accumulate goods for the sole purpose of stockpiling material wealth no more satisfies spiritual hunger than a diet of pureed foods fulfills the nutritional requirements of a robust adult.

Stress has become a prime ingredient of daily life; indeed, chronic stress has become an accepted norm. It can be logically argued that the fast-paced economic demands of the world's wealthiest nations are the primary cause for this high level of anxiety; in our opinion, however, the origins of your dissatisfaction lie in your ravaging hunger for spiritual satisfaction.

The circumstances of most people's spiritual inattention is the primary cause of their profound cosmic sleep. They hibernate like bears in winter. Limited by their undeveloped psychic senses to the restrictions of external stimuli, they are increasingly entranced by electronic technology and manufactured goods. With their love of logic, they further complicate their spiritual problems by flexing their intellects exclusively on worldly matters. As a result, their intuitive muscles have atrophied and they suffer from generalized psychic paralysis. Distrustful of the raptures of telepathy, they have bypassed its intricacies for the "privacy" of oral speech. As such, their ability to communicate clearly has degenerated into half-stated truths and awkward-sounding cackles.

Because of the extraordinary circumstances humans brought upon themselves, they have long lost the ability to fly like birds and swim like fish. It would appear they prefer cleaving to the ground like worker ants. It is as if they settled upon one grain of sand by which to experience an ocean.

Perusing these data may cause you to shake your heads and sigh in frustration with your extraterrestrial visitors. Perhaps the data instill in you an overwhelming urge to debate the details of our extraworld observations. In rebuttal, we suggest that you first take a moment to sit in a place where silence hangs her lacy curtains, that you sit in contemplative meditation for an extended time and honestly reflect upon that which is written. Endeavor to create an energy bridge of dynamic thought between your logical brain-mind and your intuitive heart-mind. Open to the possibilities of something new, a fresh point of view, a different way of looking at yourself and your world.

As you meditate, be sure to indulge in copious amounts of joy, of wonder at the delightful minimiracles that permeate your lives. Courageously explore the sweet Elysian visions that come from within. Become aware of the magnificent being of light that is the true you. As you do so, the heavy burdens of loneliness and grief you use like branches to prop up your false selves will begin to fall away like boughs in an icy forest.

Our intention is to inspire you to investigate the vast mysterious hinterlands of your Souls with as much energy, enthusiasm, and diligence as you have always given to exploring the unknown world. As you learn to read the outlines of your light-bodies, perhaps you will become as absorbed in them as you have always been with investigating the contours of the planetary globe.

You need not become sequestered like a monk to explore the enigmatic structures of Soul. You need not turn your back upon earthly pleasures. However, thoughtful prayer, meditation, and contemplation are prerequisites for maintaining spiritual equilibrium and a fully balanced life.

As Man Pollutes the Earth

Earth Mother's aching mass is calling you. She is telling you of her sorrow, her pain. Her torments are due to the anguish inflicted on her by your insatiable gorging of her luscious fruits. Centuries of frivolous self-indulgence are about to culminate in environmental tragedy. Bitterness from choices poorly made by earlier generations is forcing radical change. Now that you are in the difficult times—years of many-faceted upheaval—the wise have pause to reflect upon the past with the clarity hindsight brings.

Humanity's propensity to embrace the aggressive ways of fear has created unprecedented stress on Earth's geology. Distressful, angry, sorrowful, often violent emotions and their corresponding thought forms absorbed by the ground, water, and air for thousands of years is at the saturation point. Earth's crusted skin is in agony from the dumping of toxic wastes and toxic thoughts. Her pent-up energies are about to burst forth like pus erupting from a purulent boil. Cataclysmic events are poised to rock the length and breadth of her tortured body [see "Reflections on the El Niño Effect," page 251].

Common sense may yet hold sway—if you provoke yourselves into quick action. But you will be lost if you sit like timid mice passively succumbing to a hungry cat's imminent attack. Prepare a stout retreat: not a place to hide, but a place to live life to its fullest! Make Earth your protective fortress. Grandly defend her. Your enemy is fear. Your enemy is social, environmental, and spiritual disinterest. Your enemy is hatred, greed, anger, and other abuse. We warn you, the Dark Lords are being banished from Earth realms, and those who embrace evil will surely accompany them while Earth completes her long journey up the octaves of refined resonation.

How strange our stern advice must sit with beings who know nothing of peace, who have experienced only millennia of fear and war. We know that many of you feel fully justified in arguing for perpetuating the archaic traditions of temporal law. Nevertheless, That Which Shines Perpetual Radiance is adjusting Earth's energies to a higher level, and all negativities refusing to embrace Love's golden radiance will find themselves securely nestled in an otherworld environment, a method Universal Mechanic uses to maintain structural integrity in planets positioned at negative-positive polarity level.

On land, on water, and in the air a trail of rot follows humans wherever they go. To restore Earth to her natural state of majestic beauty, begin with the land. Restore greenery to its primal state. Rebirth the forests by planting trees. Plants are essential nutrients. Healthy plants establish the vitality of the ground you walk upon, the water you drink, and the air you breathe. Harvest the trees, yes, but with integrity, with honor. If you succeed in destroying the forests—as you seem bent on doing—life on Earth, as you know it, will cease.

With the same intent, place attention upon the water—the oceans, rivers, and streams wherein you dump your industrial by-products and the wastes of your cities. Toxic-saturated sewage ravages the health of beings who call water home.

As you restore harmony to the land and the water, the air will naturally follow, for all things are connected. In no way is anything separate from the other.

The Intergalactic Brotherhood of Light, in harmonic accordance with all masters of light, is endeavoring to prepare humanity for impending extraterrestrial contact. As you achieve a certain degree of racial maturity, you will be invited to accompany us, to reconnect with your galactic family, not as slaves bent before a tyrant's whip but as our equals. Those who awaken are being carefully groomed to assume their rightful places as conscious participants in intergalactic affairs. Although most humans are not cognizant of their state of evolving maturity, a great many are potentially ripe to do so.

Many have already reached a point of light-assimilation and are no longer frightened at the prospect of starfleet visitations. Their attraction to mysterious beings hovering in the clouds is accompanied by the realization that their energies are best served by exploring the awesome, expansive beings they truly are.

Adonai.

To Expand on Darwin

Entranced with nature's mysteries, Charles Darwin devoted his energy to the study of species' diversification and evolution of form. In the process he arrived at conclusions adaptable to the perceptions of European culture from his moment in historical time. Far-reaching in scope as they were, his deductions lacked an element of creative passion. As a grove of trees will hide a small garden from view, he overlooked certain important mystical points. Blocked by the cultural restrictions of his day, he failed, quite unintentionally, to consider an important component of natural law: Earth-positioned life forms are spirit manifesting as physical beings. It escaped his notice that a being's physical form parallels its state of vibrational sophistication or its status of evolved spiritual adaptation. He failed to consider that life is formed upon Soul- or light-energy.

Soul expresses itself over an inestimable period of time in one form after another. Eventually it outgrows the need for patterning life as a third- or fourth-dimensional corporeal being. This fact is true for plants and animals as well as for humans.

The foregoing contains broad scientific implications. Deeply significant is that there is no condition justifying a ferocious act upon one's self or any other being as is indicated by the ideology of survival of the fittest. Unfortunately, "an eye for an eye" became standard practice aeons ago when the Dark Lords assumed control of this universal sector and malevolent beings settled on Earth at the time of life's flowering. Angry and frustrated, they defiantly renounced Light's radiance—Universal Law based on the fundamental principle of unconditional Love.

Now many humans are outgrowing their need to maintain third-octave physical status. The majority are awakening starseeds, spirit beings who were implanted upon Earth as long as five million years prior to current time from various star systems. Before they were caught in the web of perpetual sleep, their Soul bodies agreed to reawaken two thousand years following the ascension of the Christ Essence, their leader in perpetuity.

As starseeds began to slip into the quaint inertia that Earth imposes upon its life forms, all but a few assumed a state of semipermanent Soul somnolence. Memories of their extrasolar origins became locked within the sorrow-filled recesses of their slumbering hearts. They rankle with unrelenting spiritual hunger. A voracious craving for Home influences every life they have lived on Earth. Circling the karmic wheel from life to life, they created a set of circumstances in accordance with that which they pledged: to wade through many Earth lives awaiting their moment to return to the stars.

All things evolve. All things seek to merge with Prime Creator. Ultimately, the whirling masses of starlight that make up the galaxies of any universe reach maximum light-saturation, at which point their entire contents (suns, planets, and so forth) begin a vibrational upward-spiraling momentum. Eventually, a bridge of cosmic matter is formed linking the lower universal densities to the resonating tones of an adjoining lighter vibration. Humming like a colony of busy bees, the heavier-toned dimensions begin to feed into the base domains of the more refined tones. Simultaneously, the harmonics of the receiving dimensions stretch to form a windowlike portal. As evolutionary universal matter maneuvers into position, a receptive doorway stretches to full magnitude. At this point the starry bodies of the entire universe, all galaxies in unison, begin to pull asunder. Assuming a form resembling a narrow-waisted wasp, the center segment of the evolving matter becomes thinner until the moment of climactic entry is reached. Celestial portions prepared for ascension begin humming at a greatly clarified amplitude as they move through the upward-spiraling energy portal set to receive them. Conversely, at the opposite end of the spectrum, with a great heaving sigh the de-evolving segment begins sloughing downward.

Meshed together like ball bearings within a wheel, life forms caught within the energies of a simultaneously ascending/descending universe cannot avoid the effects of mass cosmic evolution/de-evolution. The crossed swords of Cosmic Law in a free-will universe require every celestial body and its attendant life forms to assume responsibility for maintaining themselves in pitch attunement (at-one-ment) at each individual's level of spiritual attainment.

History, as contemporary humans fashion it, is swiftly drawing to a close. The time has come for the starseeds to shuck off the shells that have long entrapped them. They are passionately determined to return to their stars of origin. For the most part, they remain unaware of the ramifications of the multilayered events their Soul-Selves set in motion. The majority of those who fervently seek will ascend into plains of perpetual light; however, among those who were implanted, a small retinue of self-delighted beings came to Earth in darkness. Many will choose to remain in darkness.

To those who swell with pride that they are of extra-solar origin, let it be known: Opportunity for light-ascension by Earth-connected Souls parallels that of starseeded Souls. If you believe you are an implanted starseed, you must understand that many Earth-based beings resonate to this sun, Sol, as their native star. Their Souls hung like clumps of light in the ethers until it was Earth's time to experience form.

Light-Love maintains vibrations of Light-Love wherever Soul originates. One being is never favored over another. Will is the determining factor for spiritual advancement. Regardless of one's native-star origin(s), Soul matter does not deviate in substance. Soul matter is Light-Love energy extracted from the fires of creation's furnace. All Souls are light-essence quality. Soul simply adapts itself in the most practical and appropriate format for a particular planetary-spatial setting. Soul energy is Prime Energy in perpetuity. It is never depleted; although it can expand and contract, it cannot be extinguished.

Soul does not always express itself as a physical-dimension being. Generally, Soul prefers more peaceful regions of etheric light.

This stellar hum is now complete.

Human Duality

Your prolonged skirmishes with time and third-dimensional duality are coming to an end. Future's lovely pledge looms close. That which transpires will close the final curtain on unevolved human history. Like gossamer-veiled fairy tales in which everyone lives happily ever after, the rich fabric of Omniscient Being is weaving a story of everlasting joy and is spreading Its exquisite radiance around Earth's entire circumference. The theme of this exotic fable is fashioned upon the embers of hope birthed in the recesses of long-forgotten times. The stressful centuries of humanity's youth have always hinted of better times to come. In spite of all the trials and tribulations humans are subject to, for aeons the silent promise of a peaceful world has endured the scorn and derision of more-pragmatic beings.

Falling prey to duality's double standards, humans have always suffered the chill of prolonged cosmic sleep. Generally unaware that they are Soul-level-designated principal planetary stewards, they bypassed their primary obligations and assumed the role of chief resource consumers. Though humans are more than capable, even at their third-density level, of experiencing universal perfection, they are unaware that the original collective intention was to erect magnificent cities spun of finely woven gold and studded with jewels reflecting the prisms of rainbows. Although their underlying desire has always been for a harmonious existence, from childhood they are tricked into believing that a state of perpetual grace and Love's sweet promise will be boring and deleterious to their interests.

Caught in a sticky web of dualistic illusion woven by your cunning captors from the nether worlds, you were fooled into believing that you would be best served by ignoring your tender hearts' impulse to create a peaceful, harmonious society. In other words, they convinced you that Eden was not in your best interests. Tormenting you with images of an angry, vengeful god, they convinced you to blame only malicious fate for the state of your perpetually warring, stressful existence.

When a being achieves the fifth- and sixth-vibratory realms, no degree of darkness remains. When you achieve light-body ascension, you will reside upon worlds of light where That Which Is is life experiential and where the space among stars shimmers with Love's brilliant flame.

The ability to integrate unconditional Love as intelligent energy is encapsulated within your hearts in a center of to-gather-ness where the etheric DNA of your spirit body fuses with your physical DNA. The flip side to your dualistic nature is your struggle to manifest light in the physical realm—a by-product of the Law of Free Endeavor. Eventually, the balancing aspects of karmic law will pivot you into position where you will be able, in an effort of willed self-determination, to purposefully thrust Light-Love in many directions simultaneously, thus releasing yourselves from the chains of negativity that have kept you suspended in cosmic slumber. Ascension is obtainable by those who surrender ego will in passionate service to Omniscient Will. When the moment for density transfer arrives, luminescent angels will descend upon Earth and lift you high into the realms of perpetual Light.

Grace—to be held in the fluttering wings of angels—is bestowed upon those who practice Universal Law. For the most part, those who are slated to accompany Earth as she moves into the higher-octave resonations are individuals who lead quiet, unprepossessing lives. The spiritually courageous are those who are learning to transform physical mass into webs of pulsating, multihued light. As the new dawn breaks, laws that govern human society will be in harmony with those that bind all cohesive beings of the greater galactic community in integrated unconditional Love.

Pronouncements of Universal Law thoughtfully outlined in the pages of this and many other celestially inspired manuscripts pulsate like drops of rain descending upon Earth from the cloud-cloaked starships. The Law of One is easily followed. Those who will themselves to spiritually mature by practicing unconditional Love will eventually don the golden luminescence that is characteristic of a light-world being.

As the golden age settles in, it will no longer be an experiment in futility for those who live upon this planet to harmoniously sustain themselves. All who inhabit Earth will know rapturous abundance and sustainable peace as a constant life condition.

As thought energy fades, Malantor softly exits this essay's contours.

Adonai.

Regarding Suicide

Those who intentionally sweep aside their physical bodies in a less-than-idealistic attempt to dis-inhabit life are not likely to assume angel wings. Those who use suicide as a last resort to escape the despair and hopelessness of their lives will soon discover it a temporary stopgap. In most cases, those incomplete beings quickly reincarnate for another go at Earth school. Entering the astral realms, they soon discover that it is no more possible to bypass the trials and tribulations of contractual Earth lessons than it is to skip a grade in school without proper preparation for moving forward. Thus, a repeat life is in order before Soul can advance another step further on its journey Home.

In current time, the choice to exit life through the means of suicide is assuming new connotations. When the claws of disease or accident chew upon the body like a ravenous demon, and when life would have ended under natural circumstances, those who are retained in the physical against their will through the intercedence of "modern" medical technology may justifiably use suicide as the means of liberation.

In discussing suicide, we must also address the mini-suicides that many commit every day. Enervation of life force is accomplished in many ways—for instance, when purposefully ingesting known toxins such as street drugs, overindulging in food or alcohol, and taking unnecessary risks when maneuvering an automobile.

To commit suicide or not is a complicated question and is not easily addressed. At Soul level these things are approached during between-life conferences on a case-by-case basis. Simply, suicide may be considered a just cause for exiting life if life lessons are complete. Suicide is considered an unjust cause if it is used in an attempt to bypass Soul growth.

Resorting to suicide as an avoidance mechanism to override cause-and-effect consequences from inappropriate life decisions creates a karmic situation that prompts instant incarnate recall with a duplicate agenda. To purposefully vacate a terminally ill body that is being kept alive by drugs and machines for the purpose of fulfilling temporal law or the wishes of family members is reasonable from the standpoint of spiritual law. When desire for "no heroic measures" is bypassed because the agendas of family, friends, or medical or legal professionals demand it, much karma is absorbed by those who would delay another's return to Spirit.

Like butterflies deprived of their wings, the spirits of lesson-incomplete suicides hunger because their prebirth agreements contained no optional clauses for bypassing destiny. An unjustified suicidal act is serious for the Soul. Nevertheless, the Law of Free Endeavor permits not even That Which Is to interfere with individual choice—even when consciousness is ignorant of higher law.

Death is much different than most humans believe. Death brings no agony upon the spirit. Spirit body does not suffer vile circumstances unless, of course, it so chooses. As spirit exits physical body, a great sighing breath is heard, as if all the beautiful songs ever sung were celebrating mortal being's return to immortal Spirit. Physical-to-spirit transfer is like being released from a state of sluggish imprisonment to fly as free as a bird.

Death and suicide are not duplicate experiences. You may find this statement strange, but few humans understand the multidimensional aspects of death because of the deceitful beings who have duped them into fearing death. Most humans have been tricked into believing that reality is limited to physical-plane experience. Unaware of the higher realms of existence, they stumble through life without realizing that their physical selves are only approximate representations of their higher Selves. Third-dimensional experience bears little resemblance to the realities of the spiritual planes. To be surrounded by music as delicate as the breath of roses, to float upon a beam of light between the stars—that is "death" for those who face it with spiritual dignity intact. Those who transfer in a state of fear land in battlements of fear. Spirit body by itself cannot rise higher in vibration than the primary emotion it carried in life, particularly when the departing aim is to cheat destiny. To purposefully attempt to overstep spiritual law—which is the very essence of goodness—bequeaths turmoil upon the etheric body. Transposition from physical life to the Elysian Plains and back again is no more than a snap of the fingers in the cosmic scheme. As you incorporate spiritual teachings into your cognitive sense of greater reality, you will learn to rise above the impermanence of temporal life. If you would but attempt to fly like an eagle above your pain and sorrow, you would behold such beauty.

Natural healers have an innate proclivity to relieve suffering. If you are so gifted, learn to protect yourself from assimilating the consequences of another's karma. Honor the ultimate will of those who choose death over life. It is not for the average healer to know the Soul lessons of their patients, for Soul-level information is accessable only by the most spiritually advanced. Therefore, unconditionally Love all who come before you and cradle them tenderly in your merciful, gifted hands. Feed them pills of hope and encouragement. Simultaneously, refrain from absorbing their energy. Shower them with light and the magnificent courage of your own spiritual conviction. Treat them with what you have learned of the beautiful spirit worlds that await them. And when permission to speak or assist is no longer granted, rest your ministrations. Be very clear: What is another's is theirs, and what is yours is yours. Do not allow the burdens that infect the lives of your patients to become yours, for if you do, indeed they shall. There is much karmic ramification for those who meddle where they have not been invited.

Dream an Abundant Dream

Flashes of finely honed lightning streak like flaming swords through the night sky—a symbolic reminder that Archangel Michael has poised his mighty weapon high above Earth. Soon, his all-powerful sword will triumph over the last vestiges of evil. Mirroring Michael, spiritually oriented humans are struggling to break loose the bonds of the Dark Lords, those tenacious negative beings who have held Earth captive in their grip for thousands of years. Now the centuries of grief are drawing to a close. Hardly a grain is left in history's hourglass. The abundant promise of a glorious future is flowing toward you like gentle waves moving over a placid river. Those who remain on restored Earth will find themselves enfolded in the gentle arms of tranquility and love.

Do you think our writings are nothing more than a pipe dream from the quill of a mentally over-the-edge woman? Perhaps they are—if you persist in believing them to be. As you define reality, thus is reality true for you.

Those who have the courage to dream a greater dream are to manifest a greater reality. Dreamers are those who rise above the shackles of society's heavy vibration to dream of a better world to come. As we often state, we know these indomitable beings as eagles of the new dawn. They are the ones who will, one fine day, climb aboard fifth- and sixth-dimensional starships. We nurture those who persistently dream of a peaceful world with seeds of abundant hope. We sustain and encourage them to find the courage to persevere. We treat them to a starry banquet of Love. In time, they will feast their eyes upon a lush, vibrant Earth environment.

We shall meet face-to-face, and together we will explore the stars. This is our pledge to those of you who are endeavoring to evolve. Although you may believe we are outrageously unreal, the truth is that our presence is not newly recorded in these documents. Extrasolar telepathed messages can be found in the so-called legends of Camelot, Atlantis, and Lemuria. Faces of "gods" from the stars are outlined in Greek, Roman, and Nordic mythology. Portraits of your starry ancestors are carved in intricate glyphs of Mayan pillars, in stern-faced statues on Easter Island, and in haunting images of the "gods" of India and China; embedded in the prophetic teachings of the Hopi Come Home and aboriginal Dreamtime; and encased in megaliths strung like pearls around the English and French countryside. Earth is rich with clues of our existence, yet stubborn humans refuse to acknowledge us.

As the troubling years of the twilight times draw to a close, the sacred knowledge of indigenous peoples will be respected. Many so-called primitive peoples interacted with star beings, usually through the shamans of their tribes. Early peoples had extraterrestrial assistance to erect carefully positioned carved stone pyramids, arches, and domes. The sacred literature of all ancient peoples is ripe with stories of extraterrestrial visitors and the teachings they brought with them.

What was, is, and what is, was. Wherever you wander you have already been. Mystery of mysteries, the Earth holds her own.

It is anticipated that these verses will ring in your mind like the chimes of a crystal bell. May they hum melodiously in your intuitive mind's ear.

Adonai.

Spiritual Fuel

Your Self's overpowering longing to return to Universal Soul Home is the same mechanism that triggers your procreative urges. Unfortunately, your insatiable desire to be One with God is often misconstrued as an overwhelming desire for sexual coupling. Confused by your instinctive passion to self-replicate, most of you do not understand that your underlying motive is to reunite Soul with God. In many, the burning passion to establish short- and long-term relationships is motivated by sexual attraction.

Impulses that spark your body's physical preparations for sexual coupling can be compared to propellant for igniting your vehicles. The dichotomy, however, is that individuals who, for whatever reason, feel it necessary to stifle their natural needs for sexual release put themselves in danger of suppressing life-force vitality. Paradoxically, those who are subconsciously spiritually desperate often overindulge in sexual activities as a means to offset the pangs of their severe hunger for God-realization—an unfortunate situation that often finds them idling on their last drop of life-sustaining fuel: prana, or chi.

A sense of being disconnected from Source Generator rages at the center of nearly every human heart. Although positive self-discipline attributes are of primary importance for serious spiritual practitioners, the passion to merge with God is not unique and the ability to accomplish same is certainly not reserved for the spiritually adept.

All Earth's creatures must have an adequate supply of food, water, shelter, and air to sustain life. Humans, seeking something more than basic necessities, persistently distract themselves with the allures of material-based technology. Consequently, they are on the verge of accomplishing worldwide vital-resource depletion. The inevitable outcome would be mass species suicide. To reinvigorate physical, emotional, and mental maintenance, they must soon supply themselves with a full tank of spiritual fuel, that is, baseline cosmic energy. If they continue to resist nurturing themselves as spiritual beings, soon they will completely deplete their reserves.

The majority are so engrossed in transitory physical pleasures that the hum of their Souls' dream whispers at a sound-depressed point. For the most part, humans have become incapable of manifesting greater purpose in third-dimensional reality. Their deep yearning to light-activate is ravaged by the insatiable bloating of their self-consumed, spiritually starved society.

In humans, the Memories lie dormant while remaining demonstrably apparent in their dreams and meditative visions. Only briefly glimpsed and vaguely understood, the Memories surface as illusive, intangible, disconcerting, seemingly vital and purposeful images that persistently flash before the awakening eyes of the mystically inclined. We will clarify this remark by using Patricia's life as an illustration. She was born with the innate ability to cocreate telepathically with extraterrestrial beings of light for a specific life's mission. Because prelife recall was purposely suppressed from her conscious mind until midlife, her early years were spent in an almost-raging search to recall or rekindle something—she knew not what—that she felt she had lost. When she received a forceful Memory nudge in the transformative year of 1987, she suddenly stumbled upon a partial truth as to who she really was and why she had incarnated as Patricia. Like all Earth beings (human and otherwise) who are preparing themselves for light-body ascension, Patricia's Soul task is multifaceted. The clauses of her solar agreement are not readily grasped within the rigid confines of Earth's social, religious, and scientific belief systems. We anticipate you will understand that Patricia's difficulties are analogous to your struggles and that there are important, underlying reasons for delaying Soul-purpose activation in some individuals.

Deep meditation will assist you in perfecting a sense of synchronous timing as well as in developing your unique intuitive skills. To access Soul-level resonation you must practice and refine certain spiritual disciplines, the most important being meditation. You must become adept at one-point focus, the spark of concentrated will, to instantaneously ignite Self-Essence fuel. Activating Soul energy from a standpoint of high intention is the impulse that sets higher-purpose gears in motion.

To manifest Soul energy on the physical plane, meditate on the visionary stories that captivated you in childhood—because you were born with a certain level of Soul knowledge intact. Query yourself, "What made me the happiest, what did I most desire, when I was young?" When family and friends asked, "Little one, what is it you wish to be when you grow up?" what said you? Was it doctor, lawyer, Indian chief? The truth is, the answer may have been so intensely personal and astounding to your young heart-mind that you dared not speak it.

For some, childhood's dreams remain clear throughout all of life, even unto the completion of the temporal body's journey. As they transform into adults, many eagerly manifest the treasures of their youthful fantasies—a beautiful thing to behold in those who are able to clearly distinguish the beats of their inner drummers. For most it is not so simple a task, and the struggle to know themselves is pursued with great difficulty.

As the rhythms of evolution's song sweep Earth clean of karmic debris, the awakening are increasingly motivated to remember themselves from the standpoint of Soul identity. They are passionate for higher knowledge. They are consumed with desire to activate life purpose. Memory-enhancing devices such as books and movies are increasingly available to help you prepare for extraterrestrial contact and light-body ascension. For instance, the purpose for publishing Patricia's Arcturian-inspired books is to provide cosmic teaching manuals that outline procedures for attaining galactic citizenship.

When you have clearly stated your commitment to serve Soul's higher purpose, you must dynamically and purposefully pursue the aspects of your life's special mission with vigor—and it will undoubtedly require a great deal of effort and courage to do so.

Earth is a primary teaching planet. As such, she is rich with spiritual opportunity. As Soul, you ventured from the higher planes to experience the many challenges Earth's physical status has to offer. To broaden the scope of your current level of self-awareness, make a conscious effort to be aware of the beings of majestic light who are your guides and etheric support systems. Learn to keep yourself tuned to the harmonics of their refined vibrations.

Be clear about the adventure of awakening. Boldly, determinedly, and courageously forge ahead. Become a citadel of spiritual strength, a bastion of goodwill, a fortress of right thought and right action. As an eagle of the new dawn, you are enlisted in Michael's Legions of Light. As such, your mettle is being tested. Your thoughts and actions are being monitored. Tedious as this may be, stay solidly planted, firm and unyielding in your commitment to personal and planetary evolution. Be a center of peace that less-resourceful beings can rely on during the tormentuous years. Steadfastly refuse to participate in the deadly game that the Dark Lords are playing in a last-ditch effort to snare the unwary.

Peace of Mind Is Simply Achieved

Spontaneous, intuitive inspiration requires little effort. The melodious song that Self sings comes forth with little prompting, like an eagle lazily stretching its wings. Make time for your creative juices to flow. Capture and record your inner images, those brief moments of insight that bring you so much personal satisfaction.

There are many ways to prepare yourself for inward communication. One very effective method is to sit still and chant *Aum*. One note held with concentrated intention has the ability to promote within you the vibrational hum of Divine Intelligence. Although you may find the complex weavings of a Beethoven symphony more alluring, the simple sound of *Aum* contains a cosmic rendition of miraculous life.

An undisciplined brain is a feeble brain. Waves of thought are overwhelming and limit your ability to remain calm. Cacophonous inner noise is as much a physical insult as is cancer. When the brain is never still, turbulent thought gives one little peace of mind. Confused humans allow their minds to dart from issue to issue as they chew upon one bony thought fragment after another—back and forth, back and forth. Their disruptive mental chatter causes them much emotional distress and can lead to an onslaught of disease, accident, or psychological disturbance.

Internal serenity is conducive to exterior calm. Mental tranquility is a by-product of routine deep meditation, quiet moments when the mind is kept purposefully still. Disciplined thought makes gentle waves and flows peacefully through the mind. Disciplined thought rises and falls like soft breathing when the body is at rest.

Learn to erect a mental bridge to intentionally link your thoughts. Allow your mind to bring forth in beauty. Your mind is an artist. Paint majestic pictures with it. Use creative-visualization techniques and affirmation exercises to open your intuitive eye, to strengthen your neural receptor-senders, and to invigorate the mental-energy pulses your brain transmits to your body's tissues and organs.

For the uninitiated, maintaining a consistent state of meritorious thought requires supreme, concentrated will. Training the mind to properly function is no different from honing the muscles for peak performance. Effort must be vigorous and consistently applied. You will know you have achieved peaceful harmony of mind when you can insulate yourself from the powerful, distractive waves that undisciplined minds are always projecting and overcome the persistent nagging of the false ego's voice.

Peace is born in silence. Unrestricted mental energy is as disturbing to repose as are the sounds of a jackhammer tearing at concrete. Endeavor to soften your thoughts until they become as light and fluffy as drifting clouds. A disciplined mind is a sharply acute mind. Focused thought is fundamental spiritual building material.

There are no complicated guides or rules for meditating. Nevertheless, the practice of routine meditation is an art in that through its creative use it is possible to move purposefully through the universal levels and simultaneously attain Soul bliss or ab-Soul-luteness of Being. Meditation is the primary spiritual tool of choice for those who are preparing for light-body ascension. The spiritually ambitious are urging themselves to perfection, a state of being that can be achieved only through diligent efforts to establish harmonious inner peace.

Hush now, and join Malantor in song.

Hum softly the notes of the celestial Song Universal: Aummmmmmmmm, Aummmmmmmmm.... Still, the heart in rapture doth fly.... Aummmmmmmmm.

Earth

Earth's physiological requirements are duplicated in the blood and perspiration that heat and cool the human body. Earth's vital organs are supplied with life-force nutrients through streams of liquid magma that move through her veins. Streams of planetary blood originating in the beating rhythms of her core (heart) pulse upward, downward, and from side to side. Rivers and streams cool, lubricate, and flush excess heat from her tender skin. It may appear that streams of water and magma only meander; however, their courses are purposefully laid out.

Consider Earth's respiratory system—the swirls and configurations of ever-circling air. Attempting to remain oblivious to the stench that rises from their industrial wastes, humans appear to nurture a propensity toward suffocation, for they are seemingly bent on inhaling a bewildering array of toxic gases they are forever releasing into the once-pristine air. Flowing skyward, noxious pollutants tear at the delicate spatial cords that connect Earth's spirit body to the greater celestial hum.

Earth Mother radiates vibrantly. She is planetary life essence. She is beautifully clothed in a canopy of butterflies, serene mountain pools, forests, vast grasslands, herds of buffalo, great cats that creep over rocks and through thick underbrush, and birds whose exuberant voices fill the ether with song. Alive, alive is she! Sadly, contemporary humans, particularly those dwelling in huge cities, are so engrossed in their personal busyness that they are virtually numb to the subtle rhythms of Earth's planetary hum.

Dare to awaken! Dare to call forth the thunder and lightning of intensive enlightenment! Dare to shatter the tight chains that bind your Soul to spiritual inertia. Warm your stiffly held shoulders with beams of self-other compassion and unconditional Love. In meditative mode, gather bundles of roses and ferns and reflect upon their beauty. Use this imagery as a doorway into the depths of your hidden self. Understand what a great privilege it is to be granted physical life upon a world as young and vibrant as Earth is. Simultaneously, be alert to the rapidly maturing planet, for her quickening is at hand. As a resident of Earth you cannot escape her cosmic destiny. Learn to observe her from a higher perspective, as if you were monitoring her from the observational portals of a starship. Become extrasensitive to the swirls of spatial energy that periodically engulf her in preparation for her celestial event. Align yourself with the thousands of awakening humans who are aware that the entire spectrum of her diverse flora and fauna is being positioned to move either forward or backward in cosmic time.

Humans must now acknowledge the existence of less-noticeable creatures, such as small humanoids who, several centuries ago, went underground to escape the furies of their taller two-legged cousins. Do you know there are wee people living underneath your streets, lawns, gardens, and trees? Fairies, gnomes, and like beings are intelligent, astute creatures, yet most adults dismiss them as illusionary fabrications from the minds of bookish dreamers, by-products of overactive imaginations, extensions of childhood fantasies.

Are you aware that some of the most evolved minds on the planet are ocean dwellers? Did you know that dolphins and whales were originally transported from the star systems of the Pleiades and Sirius or that these highly intelligent sea creatures volunteered for Earth assignment? Not recognizing their true worth and unaware that the magnificent cetaceans are their extraterrestrial counterparts, humans launched what amounted to a full-scale war upon their gentle sea cousins in an effort to eradicate them. Ask yourself, Would I be willing to sacrifice my life's blood by volunteering to be trapped in a fisherman's net or to submit to the thrust of a harpoon for the sole purpose of enlightening my tormentors?

One of our missions is to instill insight in those who indulge in carnage of nature's simpler creatures. We find this a complicated task, for these individuals are generally too self-absorbed to pay much attention to the intricate needs of other-than-human beings. The damage their insensitivity inflicts is immature and irresponsible. The environmental discord left in their wake has become so pervasive that, even with the greatest urgency, good intentions, and state-of-the-art technology, humans by themselves are no longer capable of reversing the sorry trend of ecological malfeasance.

Beings poised for ascension into fifth- and sixth-spatial resonations include the mammals who inhabit Earth's oceans, courageous creatures who have always endeavored to live in peace and harmony with humans. In spite of the efforts of well-intentioned people, at their current rate of decline many species of whales will soon become extinct. Eradication of whales will be not from natural causes but from humans' unscrupulous behavior. If whale depopulation is successful, and if whales choose not to reestablish in this spatial sector, interaction with whales in the future will require a journey to their home stars.

Earth was designed by Prime Creator as a multifaceted jewel, a grand tapestry where the art of embellishing diversity of form could be explored; thus, the configurations of this essay are heavily sculpted. It is a grave thing to scour a planet clean of life's intricate details. It is difficult for us to understand why humans permit themselves such liberties. In their eagerness to strip Eden bare, humans have become interlopers, trespassers upon the rights of other creatures great and small. There is no honor in causing other beings to cringe in fear. Although they are nature's principal custodians, most humans have set themselves apart from her. The way that they treat Earth is as if they were to take razors and tear at the hair and moles of their skin or to immerse their hides in vats of toxic waste.

For our part, we have assumed the role of alert parents who keep salve and sterile dressings at hand to aid beloved children who insist on playing dangerous games. But evidence of imminent environmental collapse should be obvious to even the least astute. This is becoming increasingly serious, for those who choose to ignore the karmic ramifications of planetary devastation are making it more and more difficult for those who are endeavoring to prepare themselves for integration into the greater galactic community.

You who awaken welcome our assistance. We know this. Our work is greatly facilitated as increasing numbers master the technique of silent communication. By day and by night the thoughts your awakening minds project toward the stars are monitored. They drift like dancing flowers into the starships' crystalline recorders. Ripe they are, sweet and ready for plucking. You are the intrepid ones, the eagles of Earth's new dawn. Your perceptions of the universe and your rightful place within the galactic community are irreversibly changing with your growing knowledge of multidimensional reality.

Earth has always been closely observed by beings of light from a multitude of stars, galaxies, and alternate universes. Although we are quite capable of instantaneously restoring Earth's surface to pristine health, the primary obligation to do so lies with humans, and it is the responsibility of those who govern to set things in motion. It is the responsibility of the masses to see that they do. It will not serve your interests to wait until tomorrow to begin. In all frankness we must caution you: There are very few tomorrows remaining.

You query us, "How is a massive campaign to restructure society and purify Earth Mother to be logically carried out?" We respond that the methods are clearly written in many books and are basic to the teachings of all sacred literature. Investigate these resources and put into meaningful practice what is discovered. Be still and listen to Earth's lovely song, for its quiet intensity should be sufficient to stir into action even the most resistant.

The Dissipating Veil

Patricia easily communicates telepathically with beings of light, though her (third-octave) placement and theirs are situated upon parallel planes of reality or alternative dimensions. Most humans are incapable of recognizing the proximity of ethereal beings because their perceptual blinders prevent them from doing so. Now the webs of energy that separate third-dimensional from fourth-dimensional substance are beginning to loosen. As the veil between us fades, the spiritually alert are becoming aware of the presence of multileveled beings. Their lives are becoming profoundly affected by the universal wisdom they are receiving from their ethereal contacts. And to their amazement, they are discovering that we are all very much alike, which has a tendency to both fascinate and repel those newly initiated in the telepathic arts.

Whatever opinion humans hold on mysterious matters, it remains that the veil between us was built from fragments of illusion erected long ago by less-than-honorable beings who convinced their slumbering human captives that a trick of fate (documented as original sin in the Judeo-Christian Bible) was responsible for permanently separating them from the Godstate realms. Now that the slumbering phase of human history is ending, soon even the least observant will not be able to ignore the parting of the veil, for its presence is about to dissipate altogether.

Traditionalists view "death" as an impenetrable curtain between the material and spiritual planes—a separation so solid it might as well be erected of mortar and brick so thick that no living being could ever hope to visit "the other side." They do not remember how their spirits became trapped when Now time was split into three parts: past, present, and future. Nevertheless, since the beginning as humans know it, the records of all civilizations have contained testimony as to the comings and goings of majestic beings from the stars.

Contemporary scientists, in spite of their inquisitive personalities, refuse to publically initiate intelligent research into the "extraterrestrial question." Faced with a growing popular belief that Earth is being visited by "aliens," spokespersons for governments, the military, and the intelligentsia remain steadfast that any evidence pointing toward extrasolar life is a hoax. Those who stand tall and insist they have had one-to-one encounters or telepathic conversations with UFO occupants are looked upon as fringe cultists or mental incompetents.

Solemnly and patiently we await your awakening. We are rapturous as we observe the growing numbers who purposefully rouse from sleep. Joyfully, we anticipate our mutual connection. Ignoring critics and doomsayers, you who correctly intuit our presence and benevolent natures stand enraptured before the presence of cloud-formed starships. Many are also able to identify us by vibrational name and star of origin. Oh, such joy! The long Earth night is drawing to a close. The dawn of a sunlit future is radiating flames of light—flames burning the barricades of resistance that have kept you separated from your star family. As your final vestiges of sleep dissipate, we watch over and guide you from our airy perches.

Many are curious as to the nature of our tasks associated with veil dissipation—one of many functions related to Earth's evolution. An important task that has occupied us of late is the maneuvering of stone edifices you perceive as virtually immovable, such as the Pyramid of Giza. Because you are limited to measuring with rods, sticks, and the like, we find it difficult to explain using your mathematical concepts the manner in which flows of cosmic energy are subtly altering the vibrational ratios of principal monuments, mountain ranges, and other wonders of the ancient world. It is difficult because the means of construction and the primary uses of these structures (which only appear to be randomly scattered over the globe) have been kept locked away from humanity's hands until the time of cosmic maturing. For instance, in ancient times, the primary function of Stonehenge was as a stargate between Earth and the Orion star system. Orion is a jumping-off point from which various galactic segments integrate and form an opening into alternative universes, popularly termed a "wormhole."

Although many loudly insist to the contrary, your provocative imaginations desire to uncover secrets of mysterious places. Captivated by the allure of discovery, humans are always probing ancient monuments and artifacts, hoping to uncover a fragment of illusive information. Now unbelievable extraterrestrial entities have the audacity to tell you that what you are just beginning to ascertain is fundamentally incorrect. Be that as it may. We will continue to fine-tune the vibrational hum of ancient stone monuments, which, for the most part, remain highly activated structures.

We are aware our next statement has the power to frustrate you even further, but we must continue what we have begun, for this essay is not yet complete. Patricia's writings will reveal little light on the magnitude of information stored in ancient monuments and other sacred sites, for she is not privileged to unveil these profound secrets. A superbly talented individual, one gifted with psychic sight as well as technical orientation in the cinematic arts, is assigned to this project. Patricia's function is to plant galactic seed thoughts, outline the parameters of Universal Law, and set forth contractual negotiations for establishing Earth inhabitants as functioning members of the galactic core.

The thought energies of this transmission are sent forth in Love. They are engulfed in showers of radiant solar light.

Cut the Umbilical Cord

Be still, Patricia, for the substance of this transmission begins. You, too, intrepid reader, reach into the quiescent depths of your being and become as docile and as placid as water gently eddying around a submerged rock. Allow the soft, swirling image of water to guide you into the innermost recesses of self, that place which is absolutely aware of Self's connection to God.

Gracious ones, we who visit Earth do so for many reasons. One of our primary joys is the satisfaction we derive from showering your awakening minds with tidbits of celestial knowledge. Although telepathic interchange with multidimensional beings is not necessary for ultimate Soul evolution, it does enhance it, for it helps you recognize and identify realm-level vibrations. As we sow seeds of enlightenment within you, we, too, reap the stars at a rapture magnitude greater than we have heretofore experienced.

We are aware of the whys and wherefores of Universal Oneness, and we are not oblivious as to who we truly are.

We full well know the destination of your Soul journey. Another of our missions is to apprise you of the escalating flows of cosmic energy that are sweeping through the multidimensional spatial folds of this galaxy, energies that originate in an adjoining universe. They are so powerful that ultimately they will redefine and reintegrate all celestial structures within this universal segment in their transformative rhythms.

Unaware of the great cosmos that lies outside their limited frame of spatial reference, humans are virtually tethered to Earth like unborn babes fastened to their mothers' wombs by their umbilical cords. The karmic Law of Cause and Effect, the base impulse for establishing third-dimensional gravity, holds Earth's impatient offspring tightly to her bosom—an arrangement that well serves the evolutionary advantage of both humans and Earth. Humans are physically and emotionally bonded to Earth because the warped energies surrounding her girth tie them to her in a repetitive birth-death situation. Earth also provides a plane of mutual opportunity for humans to assist her—and she them—in accessing ultimate lift-off for entry into higher-level resonations.

Determined to captivate her fragile charges with her majestic splendor, Earth Mother captures your hearts and beguiles you with her awesome beauty. You, the progeny of her fecundity, are silhouetted like paper dolls before the breadth of her skies, the depth of her oceans, and the landscapes of her continents. You have become so mesmerized with her allure that your emotional and physical well-being exactly mimics hers: you are insubstantial shadows of Earth's greater being.

If your goal is to maneuver freely throughout the star fields, you must first escape Earth's gravitational pull. To do so you must disencumber yourself of all karmic debris. To regain conscious Soul Memory knowledge, you must march forward into Soul purpose with nary a backward glance when lower self and others attempt to intimidate or dissuade you. To achieve unconstrained movement along the space cords, you must first unfetter yourself of the chains of past-future time. To evolve your physical body into one of light and reestablish the sublime innocence of Soul's purity, you must make a concerted effort to develop one-point focus and be clearly intent upon your desire to progress spiritually.

Conceptual means for transforming a physical body into one of light is not easily implanted in minds resistant to such wonders. To overcome these tendencies, go gently inward and absorb these essays in a meditative state. This will help your logic-loving brain to comfortably digest their contents. Learn the rhythm of your heartfelt Soul hum until you can easily duplicate it at all times.

We are not unaware that residing as you do in third-dimensional time, it is difficult for even the most spiritually astute to attain light-magnitude transfer. For this reason, embraced within the lines of this essay are vibrational imprints that, as you accept and activate them as truthful renditions of Self's higher knowledge, will further your awareness of Universal Order. Cosmic data are interwoven as filaments of light within these essays to elevate your energy bodies (physical, auric, emotional, mental, causal, and so forth) to levels of resonation so refined that they are quite beyond the capabilities of the human mind to imagine.

Go Forth Boldly

Purple-tinged clouds glide before our starships. Dawn leaves little trace of night's shadows. As she prepares herself for ascension into the celestial realms, Earth Mother luxuriates in the dew-sprinkled light of a new day.

You who are the bravest of the brave, the starseeds, the eagles of the new dawn, comfortable in your awakening experience of Earth Mother as a living entity, stand poised upon the brink of an extraordinary evolutionary event. You are one of many who go forth onto future's path with joyful anticipation. Therefore, do not nurture yourself with visions of doom but with delightful images of Earth decorated with fields of gaily colored flowers. Garnish this image with a heavenly halo of violet light. Then fill yourself with childlike delight at what you have created. Develop this inward picture until it shines with photo-image quality. You who hold this vision are composing an outline of a powerful alternate reality, a future full of vitality's promise, one that has no room for discord or death.

Begin your task of transforming Earth's future by envisioning the sun sinking sublimely into night's crimson aura. Bask in the silence of the day's fading light. With insight acuity and focused intent, allow wings of golden light to unfold from your back and, without hesitation, go forth in earnest to become one with the red-orange rays of the setting sun. Become one with Earth's majestic star. Allow its soft brilliance to lighten, restore warmth to, and heal the contours of your wounded heart.

Practice energizing your third eye. Anoint it with oil and move the index finger of your dominant hand in a circular motion to gently awaken your dormant sacred sight. Do not lose hope if you are spiritually attuned but find it difficult to draw psychic mental pictures, for whenever you go forth in hope, your sixth sense will know you are preparing yourself for light-body ascension.

Be still in heart and mind. Move gently through your days. Dare to awaken your sleeping potential. Experience the ecstasy of merging with the sacred, with That Which Is Divine.

If you are uncomfortable with these transcripts, feeling perhaps that they contain sacrilegious undercurrents, we urge you to expand your perception of the Omniscient One. Do so until you recognize Divine Light shining forth from everyone and everything. Expand your limited perceptions until your life becomes an abundance of miracles. Psychic sight is not the prerogative of saints, prophets, and mystics. Anyone can see and know God. That Which Is is observable: Look up, there It is in the twinkling stars; look down, there It is in the scramblings of ants.

Go forth boldly into life. Become as valiant in service to higher good as was an Arthurian knight. Pledge your sword, your life in service to God's Mighty Will. Steady in stance, stay focused upon your intention to assist in manifesting Divine Plan on Earth. May your resolve to do so shine like a bright lamp turned to full-wattage power.

Our thoughts spread quickly through the lands, before the bewildered eyes of a people that barely believe we exist. We care not a fig for the lack of satisfaction that assails the masses who structure reality's form in whatever fashion they deem most suitable to their flitting desires. Let it be known: We are deeply committed to our longstanding pledge to assist in the celestial maturation of Earth's spiritual-seeking citizens.

Go forth like a hungry tiger stalking its prey and hunt down the essences of your personal truth. Never daunted, aggressively persist in your goal to break the chains of resistance your lower ego holds over you. We state once again: It is within your power to achieve light-body ascension in this lifetime. And as you will it of yourself, you become a full-fledged partner with the brotherhoods of light in a massive effort to revitalize Earth and restore peace to a people who lost it aeons ago. We are entering the final phase of this solar sector's harmonious alignment with the greater galactic hum. Transformative energies sweeping over the planet are being encompassed in the cellular biorhythms of all Earth creatures. Plants and trees bend to the pulsing rhythms of the incoming cosmic tide, for they gladly assumed the task of weaving a garment for

Earth to wear at her graduation ceremonies. Mother Earth yearns to be as well-groomed as any light-body planet as she moves into the soft flows that are indicative of the refined celestial hums.

"Chance would have it." What an interesting remark! That which humans ascribe to the functions of Lady Luck is nothing more than their minds' ability to manifest upon the physical plane. Always an act of cooperative interaction, Divine Intelligence creates that which is perfect and purposeful. Therefore, no thing enters your life by accident or coincidence. Each thought you think, each stride your body makes from moment to moment reflects an expression of your will. Though it may appear that often you work at odds with yourself (and by inference with God), the fact is that mechanisms energizing your life are activated in agreement with the expressed intention of your conscious and subconscious minds. Be very cautious in what you think, say, and do.

In addition, you must understand that your thoughts manifest as form in the astral regions prior to becoming reality in the physical realm. Thought is not limited to the brain's computerlike programming functions. The planetary airs are full of harmonic and disharmonic thought byproducts that issue from the brains of Earth's cosmically unaware inhabitants. Electromagnetic thought and emotional residue float in and out of the gases surrounding your bodies, which maintain the ill at ease in a state of constant struggle. You who awaken, endeavor to remain ever mindful of what you are thinking and what you are doing, for your evolving system is acutely sensitive to the erratic energies that less-astute beings nonchalantly toss into the ethers. You must learn to keep yourself emotionally and mentally balanced or you may suddenly find yourself squashed against the body of another person, bruising your arms and legs on tables and chairs, or, in extreme circumstances, even impacting your automobile against a brick wall.

Harmonic notes that are yours to play with in life were finely tuned and orchestrated before your birth. Before entering your mother's womb you agreed to a prenatal contract that you formed with your higher Self. Practically speaking, your prebirth Soul covenant became tremendously complicated when you awoke to find yourself caught in the Land of Nod's karmic webs. The Law of Free Intention mandates that you have the option to continually refine, edit, and rewrite the clauses of your prebirth script. The basic plot will unfold more or less in the manner your higher Self envisions, but the minute-by-minute decisions are made by your essentially unconscious lower ego, which tends to manipulate and complicate things by embroiling you in a seemingly unending series of "personal stories."

Not one to fall into despair at the tricky nature of third-dimensional energies, Soul remains cognizant at all times, for your Self dwells in plains of cosmic clarity. Your lower self, for the most part, is kept busy poking you with multilevel discomfort in its attempts to urge your "conscious state" to follow the path of least resistance. This is a difficult task, for humans are stubborn creatures who are always straining and struggling to keep a barrier in place between their lower selves and their higher Selves.

We recommend the following exercise for those desiring conscious interaction with their higher Selves. Set aside time each day for routine silence, rest, meditation, and prayerful contemplation. Create a peaceful environment using soothing mood enhancers such as candles, aromatic oils, incense, flowers and plants, recordings of soft music or nature sounds, chimes, and trickling water. Comfortably situate your body and slow your life-sustaining breath. Slowly flutter your eyelids closed, quiet your thoughts, and drift into the depths of silence. When you are physically still you open a pathway for your intuitive mind to access the telepathic cords that link you with your higher Self. As you develop your ability to listen to silence, you will eventually touch upon an ecstatic, quiescent, blissful state that is your experiential connection to Omniscient Mind. As you become more and more proficient at journeying inward, there will come a time when you will be able to free yourself of lower-ego entrapments. As your physical being establishes reentry with the superconscious planes, you will open a doorway—a true stargate—into the realms of greater cosmos, a place where you may glide as freely as any starship inhabitant upon the sweetly scented, rainbow-hued spatial light grids. Creating strands of energy that bind you to higher realms, your beautiful thoughts issue an invitation for telepathic exchange with all minds that hum in cooperative resonance with the eternal pitch of One Mind.

As you advance in meditative proficiency (which is innately natural to your intuitive Self), you will trigger an inward mechanism that will begin to alter your body's vibrational density at the DNA level, which will broaden your viewpoint of third-dimensional reality. Then you will truly go forth boldly in life!

Fling aside those safety nets! Put on a courageous face. Remember, you are a mighty spiritual warrior! Accustom yourself to balancing precariously, as if dangling from a high wire. Elevate your emotions to a level of excitement and revitalize your anticipation for entering the higher-dimensional realms. Your body's vibrations will naturally spring upward on the harmonic scale as you use simple consciousness-expanding visualization techniques. Deeply breathe in the air of intuitive clarity.

Settle for safety? Why tether yourself as if you were an anvil embedded in stone? As an advancing spiritual being, you are among the growing numbers who are anchoring light to the planet in preparation for the descent of the Dove and the masters of light. Get a sense of the inner strength this awareness brings you. Solidify your knowledge that as Soul you are indeed evolving. Do not exchange integrity and self-respect for the smaller ambitions of beings who live by a code of ethical insufficiency.

We realize that as one of the awakening you are plagued by an urgency to step into and fulfill your greater purpose. We know that there is an insistent knocking at your mind's door compelling you to release outmoded habits and that you are having difficulties with your ego's last vestiges of resistance to letting go.

Approach life without flinching. We know you are not one to cautiously lock yourself behind the negative apertures of earthly illusion. Even if you feel somewhat awkward and clumsy in your spiritual practices, your tenacity and courage to progress will see you reaching your goal.

As you go about the myriad details of your days—work, play, and relationship interactions—scrutinize the ebb and flow of subtle symbolic energy waves that are always moving through you. Develop a habit of holding a constant vision of a better world to come. Make merry! Enjoy life! Indeed, is it not a wondrous adventure?

As you become proficient at intuitive understanding, you will learn to equalize the unbalanced yin-yang energy patterns from which Earth creatures create life, and you will learn to decipher the symbolic images portrayed by your dream-state mind. Courageously obey your heart's summons to prepare yourself for integrating the full scope of your Soul's plan for incarnating on Earth.

The Akashic Library is the cosmic databank wherein all Soul data are stored. Your task, as you put your personal house in order, is to refigure your karmic balance sheet until your heavenly accounting-ledger summations equal zero, that is, debit accumulations equalized by credit accumulations. Celestial bookkeeping may seem ponderously slow from your point of view; however, the baton with which Prime Director governs the universes is delicately poised and intricately precise. Creator's tuning fork balances the harmonics of the universal chorus in much the same way a superb artisan restores sound quality to an out-of-tune spinet. As an integral member of this grand chorus, you are a singer of the celestial hum—the music of the spheres. Your intention (effort of focused will) either sharply aligns you with the cosmic melodies or causes you to drift off-key.

The columns within the Akashic ledgers are delicately tuned. At this time, the debit-credit columns are being finely adjusted. Negative-oriented individuals, those who persist in creating warps of darkness in the light-currents that play around Earth's auric body, those who prefer to wind their way through life as destructive-based forms, will have their records transferred to the pages of an alternate planet's journal. Those who choose to stay acquainted with and follow the lead of the Dark Lords will retain the privilege of doing so. The Akashic records document the comings and goings of nefarious entities whose primary intention is to invade and mismanage planets. No Soul's Akashic accounting sheet is ever lost.

In the future, you will interact with your star relatives on a one-to-one basis. You will understand that our essences are a reflection of your own being. For now, it is our privilege to offer you sweet tidbits of cosmic knowledge whose ingredients are blended from Divine Light. We are heaping luscious galactic fruits upon silver platters in preparation for a feast made up of even more delicate wonders. We anticipate you will find it most agreeable to chew upon our fine concoctions.

This data transmission originates from Malantor of Arcturus under the auspices of the star councils of the great brotherhoods of light.

Adonai this fine day's energies.

On Starships and the Space Grid

Skipping over a discussion of the complexities of cosmic physics, of molding thought to register a style of awareness similar to the way a bat's antennae direct its flight, Malantor's pleasure is to lighten your thoughts and emotions until you feel as light as a butterfly floating on a breeze. You are encouraged to approach these galactically inspired writings from a place of inner trust and knowing that you are quite capable of integrating extrasolar teachings, even if part of you remains ill at ease with the idea of telepathic communication with multidimensional-multistar extraterrestrials. Having set the mood for today's essay, I begin.

Our principal starship, *Marigold–City of Lights*, is often docked above the continental region of the so-called United States. We must tell you that, as we observe humanity from our crystalline viewing screens, what we see is not always pleasant. Because of your increasing difficulties, it is our greatest delight to assist you in these momentous times by urging you to awaken. Though much of Earth is shrouded in darkness, the auric fields of spiritually advancing humans send streams of brilliant light skyward where they reflect off the starships and bounce back to Earth like high-beam strobe lamps. The energy bodies of those who stir from cosmic sleep sparkle like sunlight on the surface of a calm lake. Joyfully your personal cosmic guides lend you their assistance as you struggle to maintain a high-level glow. In the early stages of awakening, humans' internal lights switch from on to off to on until they learn to maintain the comfortable rhythm indicative of a thoroughly activated energy body. Dancing through space, your etheric lights create a mosaic of almost unimaginable beauty, not unlike a shimmering aurora borealis. In a real way, the scope of awakening humans who emit light is a mirror image of the hovering crystalline starships.

Integrated within these extraterrestrial transcripts are bits of galactic knowledge based on humanity's classic teachings of the one called Jesus, the Christ. He who serves to Earth's evolution is of high-quality celestial energy; we know Him by the essence title *Sananda*. Christ Essence is Prime Divine Energy for sun system Sol. He is Light's Ultimate Grace. Know this: He is gathering His angelic troops around Earth's quadrants. For the time being, we hold our ships in a maintenance light pattern above Earth; nevertheless, you who awaken readily feel His profound energies, for the archangels and beings of light are waiting close to Earth. In the lofty realms, anticipatory energies run high as the angels make ready the golden staves of their evolutionary lasers. Prior to the time of galactic transfer at the end of the end times, the angels, led by the splendid host of archangels Michael and Gabriel, will herald the descent of the Dove from the starships. We urge you to prepare wisely for that magnificent day. It would not be seemly to be caught by your own higher Self in the unfortunate position of a lazy spiritual stupor.

Swinging gently along the energy webs that connect the stars, our glorious ships sail through the boundless depths of space. We hop, skip, and jump from one honey-scented tinkling light cord to the next. Stargrids are fashioned from gossamer, dew-scented, pulsating, rainbow-lit hues of light and celestial sound, and the spaces between the grids hum vibrantly. Sweetly held as if embraced by the gentle wings of angels, our multidimensional vessels glide through the purplish blackness of deep space where whirling galaxies are used as pinpoint coordinates for navigating along the space cords.

The shafts that starships revolve around are propelled by nutrients of sound, dancing colored lights, and flower odors. Magnificent crystals running through the length of these cores act as axles upon which our chariots spin. Resembling planets rotating around a sun, our interstellar-multidimensional craft travel through space reflecting the warm glow of a billion stars.

The ships' crystalline cores contain such high-magnitude energy that human technology would deem it nuclear.

However, the power source is rhythmic pulses that duplicate Creator's energy in harmony with telepathic thoughts of the ships' crews. Beings aboard the celestial chariots play as naturally as if they were on their home planets reveling in the light of their native suns. In fact, fifth- and sixth-octave extrasolar craft are majestic, miniature planets.

How we long to welcome you aboard our starships! Our intention is to prepare you to accompany us. To do so, we reach out with knowledge so profound as to shed clear understanding upon the many mysteries that have plagued your curious minds since ancient times.

A Season to Mature

A season in which to mature is allotted to each individual in manifest reality. But popular distractions override the efforts of those attempting to serve Spirit in a manner deemed culturally acceptable. In this age of electronic wizardry, humans tend to monopolize their free time with a variety of mind-numbing, mundane distractions. In places where daily busyness is conducted, work can actually preempt prebirth contractual parameters for establishing Soul at-one-ment with That Which Is Beyond the Beyond.

Be wary of many things in your advancement to light. Yet you must make a total effort to nurture your increasing spiritual hunger. The dissatisfaction of spirit that resides at your heart-chakra level is a call from That Which Is Beyond for you to come Home. The pathway Home is clearly marked, but you must learn to read its symbolic markers. It is not enough to imitate someone else's chosen path, for to put aside Self's calling to follow a more popular way to God can create a heavy karmic undertow capable of pulling you into one of future's lower possibilities—which could prove very difficult for your Soul to overcome.

If you have just begun your journey along the spiritual path, we recommend an open-minded study of a variety of spiritual traditions to assist you in finding that for which you seek. Listen and pay attention to your inner voice, for your spiritual guidance councilors are urging you to complete your karma while your current human body remains available to you. Your quest to discover God is so profoundly personal that we cannot emphasize too strongly that you must become acutely aware of yourself as a being of light, as Soul having a human experience. Transform yourself into a knowledgeable citizen of a higher-resonating universe. Never daunted, follow your heart's voice, for it is from the place of the heart that you will discover your higher nature. From that inner place, you will be drawn to the spiritual practice that offers your Soul the greatest opportunity for advancement to light. Faithfully follow your inner voice, and do not allow another to distract you from achieving your goal. As That Which Calls is placed deep within your loving heart, do not judge yourself against others and do not settle for anything less than ultimate fullness of Self.

As you travel from your boxlike buildings, learn to routinely scan the landscape, the subtle undulating energies that waver in the distance. There on the horizon, the edge of the edge, Earth shimmers. She is poised like a moth before a flame as she steadies herself to transcend the narrow margins of third-dimensional physical reality. Listen inwardly until you can discern peals of joy that radiate from the telepathic minds of etheric beings who play host to Earth's transition to light. With your growing knowledge of spiritual exercises, particularly meditation, routinely practice raising your vibrations higher than those who are bending over backward in their efforts to ignore what is becoming obvious. However difficult your path to light may appear, as you reflect on your life you will begin to realize that your problems and difficulties are actually easing.

A time of galactic ripening is at hand. You, precious ones who awaken, are the delight of the angels as well as the beings of light who hover above Earth in golden chariots. To us there is nothing more beautiful, more satisfying than to observe a starseed stretch into awareness, to watch the first tentative, even playful efforts to discover unique packets of essence of truth. As you take the initial step to rediscover self as Soul, you take a quantum leap toward Celestial Home.

Guardians from the mysterious upper dimensions stand ready to assist you. But it is you who must traverse the spatial waters that separate us by taking one small step after another. As one who is spiritually motivated, you approach a moment in galactic time when you will overcome the karmic burdens that have kept your spirit body submerged in the depths of a lower-dimensional ocean. Do not hesitate in fear, because you will be safely guided—as long as you interpret the symbolic markers your guides place before you in their efforts to lead you out of third dimension's turbulence. If you are determined to reach a higher-octave shore, one fine day you will find yourself stepping into an alternate domain where peaceful, loving beings await you.

To uplift your spirits, we have injected into the contours of this essay on Soul maturation a sweet, underlying theme intended to seduce you into helping beings of light establish Love-Light's energy on Earth. As you traverse your chosen path to That Which Is Profound, do so as an innocent bride approaches her wedding day. When you unleash the full power of Love-Light wattage that is yours to bestow, you in fact become a microscopic mirror of macrocosmic Universal Presence.

We invite you to request Creator to impregnate seeds of Divine Purpose into the womb of your heart. It then becomes your responsibility to nurture and cherish them as they sprout into being. As you give birth to essence of unconditional Love, you will become secure in your ability to reach mature fruition as a galactically aware being.

In times long forgotten, humans were torn asunder from the oneness of Souls' genderless state. History, as present-day humans construct it, is full of traditional patriarchal prerogatives to the extent that it is next to impossible to escape the confines of male-dominated, logic-bound religious traditions. Interminable, atrocious "holy" wars carried out by all parties in the name of God will not cease until humans assume a galactically mature state and agree to cooperatively shoulder their responsibilities for Earth's well-being and for all creatures who live upon her. Long has Earth served your every need. Now, at the time of her death-rebirth, she looks to you to assume your cosmically assigned role as stewards of peace. She has turned the tables on you, and it is your collective obligation to don a cloak of humility before the new times begin. Those who willingly administer to the urgent needs of their ancient and faithful planetary parent are true instruments of evolutionary change.

These are the times Soul has hungered for. These are grooming years for galactic citizenship. Because these are the most profound times humans have ever known, do not approach them in a state of disinterest, fear, or melancholy. Become a beacon of encouragement; lift high your torch of love and light and purposefully shine it wherever you go. Ashrams and other sacred retreat centers, places reserved as revered cloisters for spiritual seekers, protected sanctuaries to escape Earth's dark energies will soon close their doors to new initiates. It has come time for spiritual students to prepare to don a dress of commonality and actively share their spiritual treasures.

I, Malantor of Arcturus, am a knightly being. I am like a squire in service to the Divine King. As such, it is my joy to radiate Source Energy. My willing service is that of a star-council coordinator representing the Regional Committee for Sol System Planetary Affairs, Intergalactic Brotherhood of Light.

Mars Probe

Planet Mars is particularly sensitive to warriorlike energy emissions emanating from Earth. In ancient times, the masculine-energized Red Planet was a hub of activity during an extensive galactic war. As a result, its surface is pock-marked with remnants of a nuclear holocaust that destroyed its sister planet, Maldek. The asteroid belt between Mars and Jupiter is all that remains of the once-proud and glorious Maldek civilization. Meteor elements from Maldek's torn carcass continue to pound Earth's cosmically sensitive physique.

Because of the severity of Maldek's destruction and the continuing struggle between the forces of light and the forces of darkness in this solar sector, emissaries from the Intergalactic Brotherhood of Light established a permanent starbase on Saturn to monitor the activities of war-loving refugees who migrated to Earth at the end of the cosmic war. Elements perpetuating the war, among others, were Orions, prelight-culture Venusians, and a small contingent of Pleiadians who were resistant to light-evolution.

After Maldek was destroyed and the harmonizing elements of Martian civilization wiped clean, Venusians' evolution was rapidly brought forward. Fourth-, fifth-, and sixth-dimensional Venus is now the principal light-center for this star system. Venus, long the primary governmental location for the White Brotherhood Order of Melchizedek, after the fall of Atlantis sent representatives of that sacred order to Earth to establish a city of light in the Gobi Desert, known in Eastern cultures as Shambhala, Sacred City of Light. Christ's brother in light, Sanat Kumara, is the primary Melchizedek emissary from the white brotherhoods for configuring Earth to starlight magnitude. Long has His element served in conjunction with the Christ Essence as an equalizing factor for permeating Earth with stabilizing energy until light-transformation of Earth's body is achieved.

After the horrors of the ancient galactic conflict, a variety of stone artifacts was erected on Mars by peace-loving Sirians, who placed them there as markers to warn Earth's peace-loving citizens of the presence of evil beings within the solar system when it came time for humanity's great awakening. When the governments of Earth launched their initial Mars probe, the catlike beings of Sirius activated a triggering device within the so-called Face on Mars to serve as a preliminary warning to humans that the legends of the fall were about to begin. Within the left eye of the Martian sphinx, a beam of elemental light was projected Earthward, where it entered the left eye of the Egyptian sphinx to coincide with the opening of the corridors beneath the ancient monument—which was erected by ancient Earthlings in honor of the noble cat people of Sirius. (The sphinx actually dates prior to the fall of Atlantis, to approximately 20,000 B.C., equivalent to the time when the creator gods of Sirius were involved in communicating and interacting with Earth's early civilizations.)

One of few artifacts to withstand the jolt of Atlantis sliding into the ocean, the sphinx maintained a sturdy position because of a gold coating that protected it with force-field energies from the wild, unstable energies circling Earth at that time. After Earth restabilized in her trajectory orbit, the coating was removed and placed in a vault upon Venus, where it awaits humanity's awakening and integration into the galactic star councils. This was necessary because the coating's energy emissions are so refined that, if left in place during history's civilizations that followed the destruction of Atlantis and Lemuria, it could prematurely rupture Earth's third- and fourth-dimensional membranes and melt the protective shield placed around Earth to protect her from Maldek energy debris.

Although Mars lost the ability to sustain third-dimensional life when the war destroyed her citizens, Venus's third-dimensional population was elevated to higher-vibrational status, though Venus's physical body will retain its third-dimensional element until the entire solar system achieves light-status elevation. In contrast to the fourth- and fifth-dimensional vibratory level of the Venusian populace, the Temple of Melchizedek in Venus's Golden-White Crystal City is maintained at sixth-dimensional octave. Because of its refined resonations, the temple is an access grid in and out of this solar sector for higher beings.

We close this essay with a word of caution: Probing Mar's surface with primitive devices and exploration teams will result in gathering inaccurate data and in extremely dangerous situations for astronauts if the scientific community does not come to terms with Mars's nuclear residue and the reactivation of ancient artifacts their exploration efforts are causing—primarily, the restoration of long-dormant extrasolar energy structures upon Mars. In addition, remnants of war-loving Orions and a small contingent of Pleiadian warriors who failed to evolve with the populations of their home stars remain barricaded on Mars. The Red Planet's proximity to Earth serves them as a primary excursion base. These veterans of cosmic wars have also entrenched themselves in behind-the-scenes activities within human government, military, religious, and economic institutions, where they manipulate humans' leadership energies for their own purposes. From their powerbase, they delight in gorging themselves on aggressively negative human and animal thought-form emissions—their primary nutrient source. Some dark beings have ensconced their energy bodies in human makeup (the Men in Black) and remain a controlling factor within secret terrorist organizations that have long plagued human history. They are masters at media and thought manipulation. We warn you to be aware of their subtle and not-so-subtle ploys. To cast over their shadowy ways, you must learn to activate and hold light within your physical bodies. Those who shine like starry beacons in the night have nothing to fear from lower-vibrational beings. Dark beings cannot enter the energy bodies of those who routinely maintain themselves at stabilized high-wattage light resonance.

Malantor, in cooperative alignment with Sanat Kumara, White Brotherhood, Order of Melchizedek, and Venus base, concludes the energy of this transmission.

Adonai.

Stone Monuments and Artifacts

In ancient times, artifacts were set upon Earth to establish permanent celestial information storage centers—extraterrestrial reference libraries embedded in living stone. In current time, their primary function is as telepathic bridges between Earth and the starships for awakening starseeds. Extraterrestrials are expanding the electromagnetic integrity of these libraries.

Buried in the mud of the Atlantic, Pacific, and Indian oceans are several extraworld structures that serve the Intergalactic Brotherhood as resonation reference points. Pyramidal in form, huge etheric crystals rest where extraworld visitors positioned them in ancient times. Starship personnel use the "computerized" chambers of these pyramids as pinpoint navigational guidance systems and to establish light along Earth's interior and exterior electromagnetic grids for vibrational stabilization of her continental plates.

Known as crowning achievements of primitive man, solid-state stone monuments were erected upon critical grid vortices. From the crowns of Earth's tallest pyramids, arcs of multicolored light flow along the planetary grids. Laserlike high-resonation light beams sweep unstable electromagnetic residue off the delicate Earth grids. We are particularly active in cleansing electromagnetic static off the grids. In future times, various pyramids, Stonehenge, Easter Island, and other sacred sites will serve Earth's evolved populace as weather barometers, or more accurately, as climate "refueling terminals" for optimal control of wind, rain, and snow. Obscure as this statement may be, initial reprogramming of sacred stone sites is underway. In the future, no longer will storms and other unstable weather conditions be triggered by negative-pulsed human thought. We are altering Earth's weather-filtering systems so that her future inhabitants may create gentle weather patterns as deemed necessary for the well-being of all—plants, animals, and humans.

Several extraterrestrial-human-constructed monuments and buildings are extremely resourceful. For instance, within the borders of the spiritually and historically rich country of Nepal is an edifice that any logic-minded individual would deem an ancient ruin, suitable for archaeological study and tourist stimulation. Nevertheless, when visiting the site, clairvoyants ascertain that hanging over the "demolished" rocks of the ancient monastery is an etheric upside-down chandelier-type pyramid, an activated funnel for channeling light. Dangling as if suspended from the sky, an enormous energy duct points downward toward the ruin's superstructure. The funnel gathers volatile energies whenever a volcano erupts anywhere on Earth. As steam, molten rock, and fire shoot skyward, a backward thrusting movement sends projectiles of highly charged energy along the grids. They gather at the site of the ancient ruin and move into and through the funnel and onto a waiting starship. Unstable energies are then neutralized to grid-receptive resonation and returned to Earth.

This essay is representative of an extraterrestrial information packet designed to broaden your perception of the nature of planetary energies. We encourage you to study primary energy to sharpen your intellectual wits as to the need to position stone monuments upon junctions of primary vortex grids.

Light-Body Ascension

The waning years of the century represent the calm before the storm. Like a blast of arctic wind, the future stands poised to tear at humanity's flimsy efforts to ward off the inevitable. Deep in the planes of third-dimensional illusion, desperate humans scramble to repair the foundations of their crumbling societies while the spiritually motivated, those who are learning to thought-communicate with extrasolar visitors, prepare for light-body ascension.

Unheard by the telepathically dormant masses, a symphonic vibrational retuning is sweeping Earth with etheric strands of harmonic melodies—an elegant rhapsody of sound. The strumming strands of the beautiful opening fugue are the introductory notes to a magnificent concerto, a glorious tapestry of tonal splendor. Brilliantly orchestrated, angelic trumpets herald the return of the Christ Essence and His flowered escort—the rhythmic pulses of thousands of multioctave starships.

We have found you; in truth, we have never lost you. The graceful rhythm of our Uni-versal (one song) Mind is Soul-level tied to all Earth's inhabitants by strands of harmonious thought.

When your intention is to ascend into the realms of serenity, you invite beings of light to accompany you on your spiritual journey. You who practice daily meditation are orchestrating sonatas, waltzes, and cantatas—musical notes that bring beams of rainbow-colored lights onto Earth grids and solidify their contact points. In meditation, practice an intentional upward movement along the vibrational scale until you have accessed the rich resonation levels where perpetual serenity is the norm.

The elegance with which you grasp the underlying tones of this essay will help link the often-wayward wanderings of your logic-loving mind to the rhythmic beatings of your spiritual heart-mind.

The seasons of Earth are moving out of the fall of the year, and the stark days of a harsh winter are settling in. Blustery winds are scouring Earth grids crisply clean. Gale-force winds as overwhelming as the sudden touchdown of a massive tornado will find the spiritually unprepared huddling in fear.

Like ants crawling up an anteater's nostril, all who practice evil's malevolent ways will be swept away. As cosmic energies flowing onto Earth escalate, foolish beings scramble for a hole where they hope to escape the inevitable, but this they will not do. Those who seek God's night side ignore the obvious and remain intent upon disrupting Earth's evolution to light. These unfortunate Souls are slated to spend many lifetimes on an oblivion-state planet, trapped in a slough of their own making. Those who traverse the path that the Dark Lords tread upon will pass through the bowels of a lower-spatial dimension until their consciousnesses are disgorged onto the netherlands of a densely vibrating planet.

Locked onto the physical double-helix DNA of humans slated for ascension are light filaments resembling nylon threads—strands of etheric DNA pre-encoded with high-resonation elemental Soul essentials. To assist you in accessing data contained in refined DNA, we urge you to practice routine deep meditation. We encourage you to radiate high-magnitude light at all times, which will transform the unique strands of your personal, superconscious energy to the compartments of your active conscious mind and overcome the influence of lower-astral visages that threaten to attach themselves to your ego-body. Emit solar-level light from your heart chakra and send forth its flames like a beam from a mighty laser. Trust your connection to your highest guides and the great brotherhoods of light who stand ready to assist you in radiating Omnipotent Source energy.

As your third eye opens and your ability to see inward escalates, pay particular attention to the visions that naturally delight you, and with compassion and powerful regard, challenge all fearful apparitions that have the temerity to appear before you. More often than not, that which tends to disturb you is nothing more than an aspect of your human personality—your lower ego—that is caught in an attitude of self-other judgment or attachment. Whenever you see yourself outside the spatial element of Now time (that is, within past-present-future time), lower ego is capable of tricking you into repeating past intonations and settling for negative future standards. In difficult situations be aware of the spiritual work you have accomplished and dedicate yourself to positive transformation of all stubborn psychological reflexes. Run a detailed, honest self-analysis. Pinpoint and acknowledge even the smallest efforts at self-modification and spiritual realignment. If you had not successfully reached a higher plateau of self-awareness, you would not be attracted to reading this book, because those who dive into multidimensional transcripts are potential light-masters. We suggest you humbly appreciate the amount of personal transformation that has already taken place.

As an awakening starseed, you were not born into your current body vehicle as a complete Soul-being. The great majority who are slated for ascension at this time came into life with a large measure of both negative and positive intact karma. Nevertheless, the spiritually motivated have the greatest opportunity in millennia to prepare for permanent light-body acquisition. To do so, it is imperative that you learn to identify the unique configurations of Self as Soul.

The four volumes that will make up the Arcturian Star Chronicles are designed as celestial teaching manuals.

Their purpose is to inspire you to strive for personal as well as planetary ascension and to assist you in reaching a point of maximum impulse for the absorption of Prime Level Light.

Certainly the proof in the pudding is in the numbers of individuals who are determined to initiate an investigative analysis of Self as Soul. There is no human endeavor more fruitful or more rewarding. Although the ability to function at peak light-performance at all times is not yet within the capabilities of awakening starseeds, there are many advanced avatars, masters, and the like who can. All great teachers invite you to use them as models of reflection, for what they have accomplished as humans is within the realm of possibility for everyone. As you struggle to evolve, reach deep inside and work on elevating your light-body energies to critical mass. This, no doubt, will require a great deal of effort on your part. Nevertheless, we encourage you to do so. Learn to assimilate and incorporate the high-wattage electromagnetic flows that are sweeping over Earth. They are easily accessed and available to all, and the knowledge of how to use them is critical in your efforts to achieve light-body ascension. Simple meditation techniques that focus on proper breathing, chakra clearing, kundalini enhancement, and light-anchoring are essential to the correct use of cosmic energy.

It is imperative to recognize true Self as Soul. Your Soul body is made up of wondrous, brilliant-hued light. We who live in the fifth- and sixth-resonation realms dwell on light-body planets that at all times resonate the bounteous blessings of intelligent, integrated unconditional

Love, Creation's Prime Energy. Self as Soul's foundation is always available to you as fuel for sustaining your third-dimensional physical, mental, and emotional bodies. Soul energy is atomic and has no qualities that can be destroyed. Soul energy resembles the dynamo action of atoms, electrons, protons, and neutrons eternally whirling through space. In harmony with Divine Creator, Soul perpetually creates and re-creates as it molds light into forms of expression. Soul is a true reflection of radiant Omnipresent Beingness.

It is not too late to prepare yourself for the perfection of essence that is light-body ascension. Most starseeds were caught in the web of Earth's intrigues many, many lifetimes ago. To unwind yourself from the bonds of gravitational karma, you must do so at the cellular and DNA level. Information encoded in the genetic strands of your spiritual and physical DNA contain a road map of ever-evolving life, patterns of energy your reincarnating self will learn to clarify when it consciously aligns with Soul's remarkable nature. Your task is to unlock the library of living light that is encoded in your DNA strands. Strive to move beyond limitation. Understand: It is only the human ego personality that does not believe it possible to experience Self as Soul.

Presumptuous as it may seem, in these times of accelerating Earth-grid energies, an eighty-year-old individual, if bold enough, has enough life energy remaining to attain light-body integration. No matter the human's chronological age, eternal Soul is ageless. Soul opportunities are available equally for all who truly desire them.

Dispense with attaching your mind and emotions to despair. Brighten your self-worth image with rainbow-hued light. Envision yourself joyfully dancing as a beam of light beneath the rays of a summer's sun. Know this: Your Essence Self, your Soul, is of starlight quality.

It would do you no harm to spend some contemplative time reflecting upon the tones of this essay, for the pages contained in this manuscript are embedded with a unique set of refined, celestial vibrations whose very essence defies human language description. Underlying resonations of all telepathic communications between humans and star-essence beings are bonded in Oneness with Divine Mind.

These are the dawning years of a bright new era for humans. It is a time when life's natural wonders will be restored. Those who intend to integrate with their light-bodies will soon find themselves before a portaled gateway to the stars. In the years of the new millennium, every form of disfigurement, all manifestations of dis-ease and heartache will tumble away. Mounds of illusionary webbing that have effectively separated humans from their star family will dissolve, and the energy veil that has kept us separated will dissipate. Then to reach us will seem like crossing the warm sands of a sunny beach. For a time, negative-oriented beings will attempt to keep a mountainous energy barrier between us, but their time on Earth is coming to an end.

Honestly query self, Are you one who has become so entranced with the tantalizing things of the physical world that you forget to take time off to visit your inward-dwelling Self? To sparkle like a bit of stardust, you must consciously nurture and integrate Soul-level light into your physical body, into the subtle anatomy of the chakras, and at cellular and DNA levels. A thorough housecleaning is in order if you wish to rid yourself of emotional, mental, and physical karmic debris.

This dissertation is base-substance outline within the yearning makeup of the song that the Arcturian being of light Malantor sings to his Soul sister Patricia.

Adonai this fine Earth day.

The Remaking of Camelot and the Kennedy Administration

Long ago there was a princely being who ventured from the Isle of Man to England to spread the tale of a submerged civilization lying to the west. His Soul Essence is well-known in modern times as a leader among leaders, having reincarnated in the form of U.S. president John F. Kennedy.

Though this startling information will find the minds of historical and religious scholars plugged with skepticism, we state unequivocally: John F. Kennedy, a man who lived a princely life in this generation, once sat as fair King Arthur of England at the round table with his chivalrous knights.

Before we proceed, we must clarify why the Soul Essence of Kennedy was slated to restore a legend that refuses to die—that of Arthur's court and Camelot. It would be presumptuous to think that an unprepared Soul would transform the thinking of twentieth-century U.S. society without preamble; thus, President Kennedy was a uniquely gifted Soul.

The Soul of the entity known in modern times as John F. Kennedy entered the Earth plane directly from the upper Arcturian dimensions, where it had been resting and preparing for a particularly difficult mission. Arcturian elders identify this astonishing Soul as "he who returns as prodigal son." This archetypal phrase is much more than the title of a classic novel or a point of reference for philosophical reflection. "The return of the prodigal son" is a word combination that emits a vibrational energy which activates a particular awakening Memory in Arcturian starseeds. Its subtle tones institute a heart-mind remembering of Soul's purpose for entering the Earth plane in times that were ancient to the ancients. Arcturian genetic material was a predominant mixture in the multidimensional, multistar genetic code blending of good Arthur and his intimate knightly circle, all multidimensional starseeds.

Soul entity John F. Kennedy, in ancient times the son of a son of a preeminent Atlantean king, trained for leadership at the height of the Atlantean Empire. At that time he was Soul programmed with information that he would be reborn in the far-distant future and hold a prominent position at the times of change, a transformative epoch that star masters refer to as the beginning of the end. He was told that at that time the human species was to undergo a cellular-genetic restructuring in preparation for establishing an adaptable multisystem race on a vibrationally evolved Earth.

Late one night he entered an Atlantean temple where he was transported through a space portal to a sacred Lemurian site in the region of present-day Easter Island.

There he underwent elevated initiations to prepare his Soul to revise the Arthurian energies as appropriate to twentieth-century United States. These energies would activate a transformative doorway and institute beginning-of-the-end energies. Leaving Lemuria, he was transported forward in time to Arthurian England, where his Soul Essence was placed in the body of a newborn lad on the Isle of Man. Early in life he journeyed to England. Upon reaching manhood, he assumed the position of king and silently maintained the Arthurian court as an Earth link to Arcturus.

By a prearranged agreement with the Arcturian star council, future Soul entity John F. Kennedy learned the craft of leadership in a country plagued with the demise of old-fashioned statehood presumptions in order to evolve a form of government that bore witness to the highest good of all people. Thus, elements of ethical change—Camelot—new to Arthurian England were brought forward to the twentieth-century presidency of John F. Kennedy.

Both Arthur and Kennedy attempted to introduce controversial, transformative legislation to a ruling class that was drenched in fear-based economic, military, and political philosophy. Because this class was spiritually unprepared to accept the state of chivalrous morality that precedes Oneness in Being in mature star systems, both Arthur and Kennedy were assassinated by those who viewed themselves as dominant. From the sorrow generated within the people, the mystical legend of Camelot was born.

Humanity is fortunate that bards, poets, storytellers, and mystics do not limit themselves to historical "accuracy." Because of them and the imaginative-intuitive nature of the creative arts, the profound inspirational beauty that was Camelot refuses to die, though many centuries have passed since Arthur's brave knights strode through England. Those who record the human story through song, art, and story voice the truth of the common people. Their sensitivity to the epochal tale of Camelot enabled them to unwittingly stimulate a beyond-space-and-time energy bond between Arthurian England and the Kennedy administration. This lock remains activated as an ethereal Earth grid running between Stonehenge in Salisbury, England, and the Washington Monument obelisk in Washington, D.C.

Historians traditionally refuse to theorize on the recurring archetypal, mythological symbolism that weaves in and out of their scholarly dissertations. Predisposed to taking a dim view of such matters, they are limited to scanning the obvious and are virtually incapable of seeing the multilayered substance of human history. Their documents fail to recognize the intuitive and psychic configurations of Earth's multidimensional levels and the interactive influence of star beings with Earth's inhabitants. Therefore, the archives that record these histories were safely stored in hidden stone vaults, where they await the beginning of the beginning.

To delve deeper into our analysis, we must first bridge an intellectual gap that exists in twentieth-century military, scientific, and political philosophy. Early in his presidency, Kennedy was counseled as to the presence of extraterrestrials, but he kept this knowledge secret from all but a select few of his inner circle. A few remain alive who remember the "odd one" that periodically came and went behind closed doors. They remain silent for fear of ridicule and retaliation. In their ignorance of the multidimensional nature of extraterrestrial activities, they simply did not (and still do not) comprehend the danger and degree of the Grays' influence in respect to pre- and post-World War II governments. Because of their failure to ascertain the role of lower extraterrestrial beings throughout human history, they were unprepared to acknowledge the presence of higher-dimensional influence in the odd one as an ambassador at large from the Intergalactic Brotherhood star councils.

Following the use of nuclear energy for destructive purposes at the end of World War II, there was imminent danger of a galactic war breaking out on the outer planets of this solar system. The remaking of Camelot was an attempt by the Regency star council to prevent this war. When the first satellite was sent up in the late 1950s, Orion warring factions again became unsettled and pushed their efforts to retain controlling status of Earth's technology-emerging nations. Knowing that Earth is slated for recovery into the intergalactic community in the early years of the twenty-first century, the Dark Lords found themselves in a last-minute effort to capture and assimilate as much human energy as possible before it became necessary for them to transfer their activities to a lower-tuned planetary vibration.

Soul Memories remain hidden from consciousness in all but the most spiritually advanced. Like all humans,

Kennedy struggled with ego urges and desires. This caused quite a flutter when it was discovered he had a propensity to womanize. Viewing his problems from an airier perspective, however, we note that his conflict (which is similar to that of all male-bodied starseeds) is that elemental creative and psychic functions are based in feminine energy. The rebirth of Camelot required an outpouring from the sacred imaginative-intuitive heart center, which required a vibrational awakening in a young lad who was psychically untrained and culturally indisposed to "such nonsense." It takes a great deal of effort for U.S.-educated males to tune their telepathic antennae to multidimensional levels.

Events associated with the Kennedy administration's official policies and procedures are not pertinent to this discussion, except to note Kennedy's cooperation with a representative of the Regency star council. Because Kennedy was open to and pushed for opening space and the first lunar probe, he established the idea that humans could move beyond the confines of their planet. In particular, he affected the young people, a generation of Souls scheduled for birth in the 1970s, 1980s, and 1990s whose life assignments would be to create a multidimensional bridgeway to the stars.

To summarize the profound information contained in this essay: The rebirthing of Camelot was accomplished through a preliminary adjutant from the Regency star council in the form of Arcturian Soul John F. Kennedy to the "United" States government to assist it to prepare for the beginning of the end. His advice and warnings were rejected by those who held positions of authority, particularly the military—the real instruments behind his untimely demise. Those who vehemently deny this accusation are those who know it to be true.

Be alert to symbolic nuances in every presidential administration since the assassination of John F. Kennedy. There has been a thinly veiled struggle between light and dark extraterrestrials since that time. It is not our purpose to illustrate who is who and what is what, but you are encouraged to take an intuitive look at world events, learn to read between the lines, and draw your own conclusions.

The archetypal Arthurian myth, in some form or other, exists in all cultures and is one of the typical symbolic means used for awakening Soul Memories within starseeded human psyches.

Nazca Lines and Time Travel

Do you believe that all ancient mysteries are connected in some way with starseed colonization of Earth? If so, you are somewhat on target. However, during certain key epochs, humankind was sufficiently advanced to sustain itself without outside assistance. This was particularly true at the height of the Atlantean civilization when discovery of an antimatter device freed a segment of the reigning elite from the need to confer with its otherworld associates in a few areas, particularly time travel. To facilitate the movement of their time-warp ships, Atlantean scientists used ceremonial sites such as temples, initiation chambers, and astronomical observatories as housing and launching facilities.

Today, developments in aerospace somewhat copy captured fourth-dimensional extraterrestrial craft. For the most part, however, elemental rocket science is strictly a human discovery. The importance of freeing humanity to evolve independently in its own unique manner without the overseeing influence of extraworld beings is an indicator that the human species is struggling to mature cosmically.

Atlantean engineers originated the Nazca Lines in the western desert of South America as assembly points for their time-warp machines, because grid energies in that region are independent of time and are capable of moving future time backward and past time forward. Virtually ignored by scientists and engineering technicians of this era and relegated to the rather limited perception of historians and archaeologists (because of the belief that past energy is dead energy), the mysterious Nazca Lines nevertheless are used by many past-future multidimensional craft to obtain instantaneous movement through the vagaries of third-dimensional spatial time. Human intelligentsia would be startled to learn how active the Nazca landing strips remain.

Humans are taught that reality is built upon rigidly established linear time lines. Only the most exceptionally trained scientists are beginning to embrace the concepts of a multidimensional universe. Because many ancient sites and monuments are time-active, multidimensionals and past and future humans (such as the Atlanteans) who possess time-energy-transfer technology are adapting the Nazca Lines and other activated energy spots, such as Stonehenge, into spatial windows, which will facilitate Earth's transfer through a multidimensional window.

The call to arouse humanity to a greater cosmic awareness, to take its place as equals in the greater galactic community, has been issued. This is the last invitation humans will receive. If the collective summons to become One within the star brotherhoods is not answered in a timely fashion, by necessity the matter will be taken out of the hands of those who have appointed themselves humanity's leaders and into those of the spiritually evolving.

Humans are treading a narrow path. In a real sense they are positioned upon a treadmill, attempting to stay balanced upon waves of escalating energies that do not stay for long on one speed but gather increasing momentum.

The landing strips quiver. Prepare yourselves. The Return is imminent.

On Purpose, Bliss, Trust, and Source Creator

Deep in the human heart beats an insatiable yearning to rediscover Soul's greater purpose. Visually adept individuals are attentive to all images that arise in dreams and meditations and use them in many situations. Succumbing to the allure of an unlimited array of sensations and experiences, however, the majority wade through life after life concentrating almost exclusively upon the physical world. They effectively block any communication with Universal Mind. Caught like flies in the sticky karmic threads of a spiritually restrictive society, their link to the Divine has become tangled in a web of vaguely understood miracles and often-frightening paranormal events.

Soul purpose is a pact Self makes with Divine Creative Intelligence before birthing into a third-dimensional body. Before agreeing to incarnate on Earth, they hold a prebirth planning session to deliberate upon blueprints for impending life. They investigate Soul's ledger—the Akashic records—with minute analysis of all karmic debits and credits. Recommendations most beneficial to Soul's advancement in the celestial realms are scrutinized. Because Soul schematics contain many substrates, the relationships and corresponding activities most beneficial to Soul's refinement are orchestrated. Then, as sperm and egg merge as one, a map outlining life's higher purpose is implanted into the genetic strands of the budding embryo.

Because of Earth's space-time placement within the third-dimensional karmic (gravitational) belt, almost immediately following birth most humans lay aside their Soul Memories, failing to remember they are eternal beings having brief encounters with physical life. As adults they become so absorbed in fingering the sweetmeats of physical sensation that they ignore the wealth of their Souls' encyclopedic knowledge. As they slide into a state of spiritual torpor, their brain-minds lose the ability to interpret the symbolic clues that remind them what they came into life to do.

Humans face a constant barrage of sensations and stimuli, an onslaught of distractions and demands by their lower selves to satiate one self-indulgent behavior after another. Attempting to survive intact on a dangerous planet, they stumble through one life after another unaware that they are directly connected to and have unlimited access to Divine Intelligence. More the pity, they exhibit little desire to overcome this Soul-debilitating situation. Frustration and restlessness are the predominant themes that emanate from them. For thousands of years they have surrendered their life energies to unremitting Soul slumber.

Nevertheless, Universal Law cannot be ignored indefinitely. In 1987, the Office of the Christ instituted a planet-wide shift in negative-to-positive thought polarities, thus assuring Earth inhabitants that they would soon be free of their restrictive trappings. The awakening are now feeling a persuasive, urgent summons to reestablish themselves as Soul energy. Though of diverse temperament and spiritual persuasion, they share a commonality in that they are integrating Soul's purpose as a primary life focus. With the flush of excitement that accompanies restoration of Divine Knowledge, they are committed to participating in Earth's dimensional shift and humanity's return to the stars.

It is not necessary to sacrifice moments of bliss for less-worthy endeavors. Whenever blissful sensations sweep over you, your serenity emanates a golden white light that pulses up and out your crown chakra, illuminating your auric body with a halo of magnificent, iridescent light. Whenever peak levels of bliss are sustained, you become submerged in the exquisite light of Divine Beingness. Advanced adepts achieve perpetual harmonious well-being and are capable of intentionally holding themselves in the blissful vibration that characterizes the greater universal hum, an advanced meditative state called *samadhi*. Now that Earth is refining her vibrational essence, the sweet condition of Divine Being in which spiritual masters dwell is within reach of serious meditation practitioners. Fountains of celestial bliss that seem to be nowhere and everywhere simultaneously are spraying

Earth with multifaceted rays of peaceful contentment, the norm for beings who live on higher-dimensional worlds.

For an individual to tap into universal levels of Divine Bliss requires an alert motivation to be in Oneness with Source Energy. This is accomplished through dedicated practice of spiritual techniques for developing Soul in Beingness. To sustain a blissful momentum, you must detach from life's down-tugging energies and surrender yourself, resembling a leaf floating along a tranquil mountain stream.

Most humans think that to be blissful is to be rapturously in love. They also associate bliss with the feelings of awe that overcome them when they view a magnificent aspect of Earth's countenance. These experiences are related to emotional bliss. On the other hand, when one achieves Divine Bliss one opens an access portal into realms where the ecstasy of unconditional Love is endlessly experienced. Unconditional Love as an expression of Divine Bliss is an integrated energy vibration. Those who dwell in Divine Bliss are snugly wrapped in the wings of angels.

There are beings with skin as blue as the deepest sea, with eyes as dark as a moonless night sky, yet their Souls' shine from their pupils like some of heaven's brightest stars. Thus we describe the advanced beings of the Pleiades. Point of reference: No matter how beautiful the exterior body, the only way to reliably identify Soul configuration is to recognize the God-Essence beauty that resides within. No matter the star of origin, in a wondrous way all beings, although remaining uniquely individual, are remarkably similar. All beings are composed of Soul, of Primary Cosmic Light, and at the core of their being, all dream the same dream of returning to Source. Although the trappings may greatly vary—the color of the skin, the physical substance, the star system of origin—Soul's purpose does not. Soul's purpose is to maintain Itself in perpetual Oneness with Source Creator. Soul advancement at all levels is predicated on an overpowering desire to move through the muted tones of the lower-dimensional hums until ultimate realm is attained—the House of the Central Sun, God's Holy Mansion.

Our human contactees, although confined to Earth's restrictive vibrations, have evolved to a point where they completely trust their telepathic links with beings of light from higher dimensions, though their human-to-human communication skills remain limited to verbal speech. This is so because humans are seriously deficient in the subtleties of mind-thought exchange. This remark should not be taken in a judgmental way. Many humans with whom we interact have the ability to clearly understand the multilevel information transmissions we telepath to them; however, because of flaws inherent in verbal and written language, it is almost impossible for them to decipher their stellar-to-Earth communications without some margin of error. Human communication is extremely restrictive; even the most skilled receptor-sender telepaths are limited by such things as learned language structure and cultural, social, and educational imprints. Because oral and written exchange between humans is so difficult, the only thing you can truly trust about others is their underlying intent and experiential perception as individuals.

Multidimensional telepathed or channeled materials are often most clearly expressed in music and art. Another area in which we interact with humanity is through our beneficial acts that compassionately and lovingly elevate the standards of your lives whenever the human heart is transfixed in harmonious rapture with Earth's natural elements.

Because individuals' language skills vary greatly, the degree of trust allocated to spoken or written words should be tempered by a self-awareness of the power of the mind to go through all sorts of mental configurations that bend and distort meaning. The heartfelt manner in which humans speak to one another through emotional contact is often much more truthful than their dialogue. When their hearts are stimulated by expressions of joy, humans are able to clearly communicate from a place of unconditional Love. Resonations emitted through qualities embraced within the core of human essence form connective fibers that link them in holy Oneness with all living things.

Those who seek God will find God. Those who do not will not. The ultimate test of these evolutionary times is for humans to learn to completely and utterly trust that they can, in all matters, rely upon Source Creator's universe to provide them with constant abundance, in all its rich and varied aspects. Those who continuously call God to them shine forth in glory, and their auras are as brilliant as the brightest sun. Those eagles of the new dawn who are taking it upon themselves to see that God's Greater Works on Earth be done are rising like phoenixes from the ashes of the unconscious masses.

For a moment, join us in meditative silence. Concentrate inwardly and focus upon Source Creator as you understand It and a particular spot within the universe called Earth. Observing Creator's good work on this planet, begin to view Earth as you know her, in her third-dimensional body. Now, allowing your vision to move upward, sideways, and back and forth, observe Earth as being made up of distinct domains or dimensional layers. Let your intuition guide you through the layers and, as you do so, realize that each layer contains a slightly different version of life's infinite possibilities. May this tantalizing vision serve as a basis for observing Earth in a new way. Perceive her as being in a state of upward-moving resonation. Now, contemplate creative Source Energy as swirling multistrand prisms of light, realizing that even as Source sends out, It draws back what It sent.

All things within this universe came into being at a specific vibrational level. Although there are many universal levels, the multiresonance layers are never separated from the energies of Source Creator.

Evolving Universes and the Octave Zone Termination Factor

Nestled like a newly hatched songbird in a warm nest, the midway point in any harmonic (dimensional octave) is best termed the neutral zone. As Divine Vibration or Celestial Sound moves through the universal substrates it rises and falls, pulsating and undulating like prairie grasses blowing in the wind. Swelling in pitch, Celestial Sound blends with Light's invigorating energies. From this union matter is born—stars, planets, moons, and so forth.

When the substance of a material universe comes into being, it enters its initial phase of existence at the grossest or lowest-level dimensional octave. From that point, Celestial Substance refines its movement through a series of vibrational or evolutionary upgrades. Intent on returning to That Which Originally Sends Forth, matter begins its long journey upward through the levels of universal light-sound harmonics. To return to Celestial Home, Creation's structures—stars, planets, moons, comets, and beings who live upon or within them—must first pass through every level within each sound-light octave.

To best illustrate universal vibrational levels, envision a musician practicing scales upon a piano, playing one note after another progressively. The fingers start at the lowest octave on the piano and begin playing by striking the lowest C. As the fingers move upward, vibrational tones rise by eight notes until the fingers settle upon the next higher C, which vibrates twice as fast, a more refined place to experience the note. Aptly put: At the point where they leave one octave to start another, the fingers are positioned at the octave transformation zone, which on the universal scale is termed the octave zone termination (OZT) factor.

The OZT is of critical importance, for the OZT junction is where the star councils strike celestial instruments that call the attributes of Universal Law into play as appropriate to each vibrational octave. As the octave harmonics of a particular universe slide into the windowlike opening that allows it to be grappled by the forces of uplifting vibrational strains, it progressively widens at both the termination end and the opening end of the following vibrational pitch, in the process becoming somewhat narrow in the midregions.

As ever it will be, free will remains for all matter, whether sun, planet, moon, or, most assuredly, animal, plant, or human. Therefore, on current-time Earth, beings resistant to octavational change—those who desire to maintain their Souls at lower pitch—are being swept into octave realms where energies that choose to play havoc with Universal Law are maintained.

As matter passes into and through the OZT zone, it enters into a region of upgrading amplitude where the internal hum of Souls dwelling there becomes refined in both tone and light. At midpoint in the lower-universal regions, those who opt for limited light or status quo vibrational status—those who prefer to seek God in a reverse fashion—are separated from beings who occupy universal hums that are sparked to become as bright as the fires of melting suns. Thus, the universe and all its galaxies and the stuff of the galaxies themselves are tugged at, turned back and forth and end upon end, so that each portion links with what is going forward and what is going backward. Periodically, universes merge matter, and above-scale harmonics absorb leading edges of below-scale harmonics.

When one speaks of a major energy shift on a universal, evolutionary scale, one witnesses routine adjustments in the harmonics of a universe's light-sound system (from our point of view, *light* and *sound* are synonymous terms). To further clarify: Remember that base-material substance throughout all Creation is made up of Source Material, that which could be likened to the body of the One. Prime Energy is derived from creative-force substance and is best described as unconditional Love, an integrated intelligence that is much more delicately refined than the human mind can comprehend. Only in deepest meditative postures (samadhi) can a human aspire to achieve holy Oneness (common-union). Then a whiff of the sweet aroma of universal honey can be recognized, although, by necessity, the magnificence of its breadth and scope will elude until Earth evolves into the light planes of higher-world harmonics.

Universal substrates evolve and de-evolve through a process of whirling matter upward and downward. Circles begetting circles in turn beget ever-widening and ever-diminishing circles. Dense material resonating within the lower-vibrational substrates is the makeup of the widest circles. The universal amplitudes in which we commonly reside are shaped like a multilayered cone made up of layers of circles resting upon circles. The lower second- and third-octave resonations circle in a continuous swirling pattern that atom particulates (dense material forms) naturally take upon themselves. Bound in place by the Law of Universal Harmonic Movement, Earth's third- and fourth-dimensional energies are bound to the balancing realms of gravitational pull that respond to base energy and are kept in proportional mode by the Law of Cause and Effect, or karmic law.

Eventually, the intense Soul desire to return Home causes cosmic matter to swirl in an ascending spiral motion, pulling all that is harmoniously adaptable with it into the escalating regions of perpetual refinement. Beings who have reached an evolutionary point when their greatest desire is to know God on an ab-Soul-lute basis are swept closer and closer to Universal Light Central, where Soul Essence eventually merges into realms of Divine Omnipresence.

In the multilayered "platter" of universes that make up Creation, our home universe's celestial energy or tonal resonation represents our uniquely individual multi-Souls (mega-Souls would be more accurate). Ecstasy of Omniscient Knowledge is contained in a mutual Soul acknowledgment that Creation's Prime Energy arises from the ab-Soul-luteness of the One.

Next to the universal layers of our multigalactic home, other cone-shaped whirling universes spin like wheels, one beside another, wheels that we who live in third, fourth, fifth, and sixth octaves perceive as formed of stars, moons, planets, comets, and other cosmic material that defies description. First- and second-degree octaves are solid and lack shape, the so-called flatlands. Third-dimensional zones offer little more. Nevertheless, the urge of life formed into gross material substance is to move, to refine, to evolve, for the pain of life flattened is exquisite.

The central axle upon which the cone-shaped universes spin is best termed Central Sun. It is from this point that Creation's magnificence moves eternally outward. Surrounding and cuddling the great mass of whirling universes is the great void—that which reaches forever outward without limit. It is quite beyond our capabilities to use human language to further clarify Source Creator's ability to expand nothingness into somethingness.

Management Training Films

It is imperative for humans to understand the origins of energy that permeates today's movies. The cinematic arts are a favorite playground for representatives of both the light and dark who are, in their own ways, preparing humanity for the end times. Movies and television are two favored fields the brotherhoods of light use to educate humans in the precepts of Universal Law, Universal Science, and the way beings of light communicate with individuals as well as with the human collective.

Cinematic art graduated from infancy into growing technological sophistication with the 1960s preliminary "galactic training film" *2001: A Space Odyssey*. In the 1970s, several aware entrepreneurs, notably Steven Spielberg and George Lucas, initiated projects designed to stimulate a welcoming taste for extraterrestrial contact and to encourage a positive look at humanity's future.

In the 1960s, another preliminary experiment began with the precedent-setting television series *Star Trek*. The visionary originator, Gene Rodenberry, is beloved by the multidimensional star councils. Prior to the series, Mr. Rodenberry was an active member of an aware group who were in contact with a ninth-level energy identified as Tom. We will not discuss the part Rodenberry played in this group; we refer those wishing to pursue the matter to *The Only Planet of Choice* [see Appendix]. Many advanced technological and philosophical ideas depicted throughout the various *Star Trek* series, particularly the concept of Prime Directive, are absolutely in line with solar science and Divine Law as practiced by higher-dimensional beings who make up the Intergalactic Brotherhood of Light.

Of particular interest is the movie *Cocoon*, an effort by director Ron Howard who, unbeknownst to himself, correctly symbolized the status of elderly starseeded Souls on Earth and their bid to return Home in spite of all odds, coupled with advanced extraterrestrials who came to Earth to reenergize and prepare the starseeds for their return.

Thereafter, many movie and television films began to depict the nature of humanity's evolutionary status, the concentrated effort it will take them to access the space grids, and the true nature of their relationship with the peace-loving beings who inhabit the higher-dimensional planes.

Aspects of evolving human potential, as discussed throughout these essays, are illustrated in popular movies such as *Powder* and *Phenomenon*.

Gray entities from Zeta Reticulum who are attempting to interfere with humanity by abducting them for medical experimentation and genetic manipulation mean well enough; nevertheless, they are operating outside the dictates of Universal Law. Because their primary motive is to ensure survival of their dying species, their reasons cannot be looked upon as completely without merit, although their methods are in question. Although the Zeta are in possession of some advanced technology in that they can access the lower fourth-dimensional or astral space-time energy realms, their level of spiritual advancement is that of slightly aware humans. Some Zeta are attempting to instruct their human abductees on the necessity of cooperative interaction—Oneness—and the dangers of humanity's disregard for Earth's environment.

This, however, does not address the motivations of ulterior-seeking beings from other star systems, such as renegade Orions who have closeted themselves with Earth's underground governments and military cartels to keep humanity under their energy-sapping control. The Orions' physical structure and motives are fairly accurately portrayed in the movie *Independence Day*. Humans' ability to protect themselves from these beings and sheer force of will to break the chains that have bound them in servitude for millennia to negative extraterrestrials is also accurately depicted, in that it must be done by a cooperative effort—Oneness.

It is important to understand that Orion is a system of polarities. Although a renegade group from Orion is responsible for much suffering in this solar sector, most Orions belong to a very advanced civilization and are members of the Intergalactic Brotherhood of Light. Orion stargate qualities are depicted in movies such as *2001: A Space Odyssey*, *Stargate*, and *Contact*.

Countless humans have pushed aside opportunities for telepathic interaction because of religious fear and fear of the unknown. From the moment we are issued a command to leave you alone—to go away—that we do. This is not to say that we desert you, only that we retire to our traditional observational mode; hence, we are often referred to as the watchers. In fact, many humans are guided spiritually by advanced extraterrestrials. Because our appearance is that of fields of light-energy, we are often mistaken for guardian angels. When you invite us again, it is then our joyful privilege to reconnect the telepathic linkages within the pituitary that unites the human mind with the collective One Mind, the very essence of beings of the galactic core.

It is imperative for you to understand the difference between challenging a contact and denying a contact. That which is challenge—"Are thee of the light?"—is imperative for humans newly initiated into the nuances of multidimensional telepathy.

We could explain the symbolic importance of several important "management training films" [see Appendix], but we prefer to encourage you to delve into your growing knowledge of the role symbolism plays in your personal evolutionary process. We also encourage careful discrimination when ascertaining which movies and television productions incorporate light vibrations and which incorporate dark vibrations. Be aware as well that there is a great deal of blending going on, for the nature of filmmaking draws many to it and the personalities of many individuals are contained within the final product. Learn to intuit mixtures of light and dark in movies and television programs. While you remain at third dimension, there will always be a marriage of sorts between light and dark, for that is the nature of reality at that level. The teachings, however, clearly point out that there is no separation between these things, for all things are of God and, therefore, are unique particles of the One, varying aspects of the Divine in manifest form.

It is critical that you who are endeavoring to ascend into the higher-vibrational energies understand that worlds are not deemed higher or more advanced because of technological achievements but because the vibrational hums of their inhabitants are held in perfect pitch with the Universal Law of unconditional Love at all times, in peaceful alignment with harmonics of Divine Light and Sound.

Galactic Management Profile

In a manner similar to slaves aboard a Roman galley ship, humans are held captive aboard spaceship Earth. Tormented souls are chained to the bowels of the lower-dimensional regions, sweating and straining from one life to another virtually ignorant of their ship's ultimate destination.

Those who captained ancient sailing vessels, those who set the course, were prepared to wage battle. The common soldiers sequestered below deck in full battle array were more or less cognizant of the general plan of the voyage, but they were not generally privy to the strategy, goals, and purpose of their commanding officers. In more modern times the captain no longer has such autonomy; although remaining observant of the seas, he must stay in constant communication with his superiors who, in turn, are obligated to keep an open channel to their commander-in-chief, the nation's primary leader.

At the galactic management level, the Christ Essence is supreme commander of all Earth-based interstellar, multidimensional forces. The Intergalactic Brotherhood of Light and its substrates, the star councils and planetary federations, serve under the governorship of the Office of the Christ and the Spiritual Hierarchy. The unified galactic management team is made up of squadrons of beings of light from many star systems in service to Divine Oneness. Prime information is received as pulses of living light and sound from a hub of cosmic activity we will refer to as the halls of the Central Sun. The brotherhoods of light—which include the Intergalactic Brotherhood of Light, the Order of Melchizedek (under the directorship of Sanat Kumara), and the Spiritual Hierarchy—are somewhat duplicated on Earth in the way the branches of the armed services form an overall cooperative league and more or less act as a unit to serve their nation in times of crisis.

For true cooperation, the system must recognize that the entire membership must be considered before any momentous venture can be undertaken. Caught in a web of intrigue woven by powerful forces in which they have virtually no control, however, the rank-and-file soldiers and sailors, who are the key element in any battle, are at the mercy of their leaders' integrity. Allegorically, you who are beginning to realize you play a role in the activities of the galactic management team on Earth do so as frontline starseeded troops. Many of you, like Patricia, endeavor to keep yourselves in a state of constant telepathic connection with cosmic command central as you receive and transmit data. Your superior officers, or guides, in turn receive instructions directly from their commander at galactic management central, the Office of the Christ. It is the commanders' responsibility to disperse information so that the guides understand the most beneficial way to disperse cosmic Light-Love energy.

The purpose of compiling celestial data in workable human form is to goad the awakening into spiritual activity. In this regard, we are forming interactive field-instruction manuals to call the awakening to arms and to prepare them for spiritual battle.

Humans who have volunteered to staff the front lines for the galactic management team are referred to in star-council meetings as sky warriors, eagles of the new dawn. For their part, Regency star-council members have been commissioned by Supreme Commander in Chief in residence Central Sun to awaken Earth's sleeping citizens to their personal, planetary, and galactic responsibilities. By necessity, the backbone of these formalities is to carry out a spiritual, cultural, economic, governmental, and military revolution by engulfing Earth and her inhabitants with successive waves of highly refined cosmic energies.

Those who choose to remain slaves of their manipulative captors, those who prefer to remain chained to the lower-dimensional planetary bowels, are members of the great hulking unconscious. Ignorant of the celestial call to arms, they sit strapped in their seats of discontent. Trapped behind walls of illusionary spiritual inertia, they cringe in hiding from their suspected enemy, that of activated spiritual responsibility.

This treatise written in military symbology is to remind you that a galactic battle has long been waged for

Earth. The stakes are extremely high, and the enemy's forces are exceedingly strong and cunning. In a real sense, the final battle to control this galactic sector has already been won by the forces of light. The Dark Lords are in the process of being tossed out of their Earth-based and lower-astral bivouacs, where once they were permitted to practice their devious ways more or less at will. The peaceful Orion elders have also succeeded in overpowering the last vestiges of dark Orion usurpers who once warped not only Earth but the lower-spatial fields of their own stargated galactic cluster. Now only a remnant of marauding Orions and their cohorts from the lower-dimensional planes remain locked within the planets of this solar system, notably Mars and Earth. They play out the last innings of their insidious game from within the safety of your moon's dark side. Along with the Grays from Zeta Reticulum, the Orions have been busy these many years harassing the unwary and absconding Earth citizens against their will. As a result, spiritually unconscious humans, who already fear the unknown, are in much trepidation as to the intention of beings who staff UFOs.

In these accelerated times, it behooves everyone to make well-thought-out life choices. The energies that have kept light-seeking humans in an interactive world with shadow-seeking humans are parting. The webs of cosmic energy that have bound humanity together throughout history are already moving along diverse pathways. Opportunity to track change is extremely limited. The decision, as always, is up to the individual.

Christ Essence is referred to in the first two volumes of the Arcturian Star Chronicles as "Sananda." Christ Consciousness is a vibrational identification given to Earth's Avatar Supreme. The Christ Essence has incarnated upon Earth in many forms, including Jesus, Krishna, Buddha, and Mohammed.

Starseeding of Planet Earth

Souls are sparks of quintessential light radiance. By nature, human Souls are lonely beings, stumbling through life marred by a lack of understanding as to the true purpose of their journeys. On the surface, it appears that their predicament is to be perpetually overwhelmed by one traumatic event after another. What they fail to understand is that although they have been manipulated by lower-energy extraterrestrials who delight in feeding on the energies emitted by humans' torments, the truth is that humans' greatest enemy has always been themselves, for humans have always had the power to break the chains that have kept them bound to their invisible captors. Perpetuating this situation, since ancient times each generation teaches its children that confrontation and aggression are necessary facts of life. Even the youngest are taught the preposterous notion that powerful nations can rise only from a culmination of factors based on solidly entrenched governments, military war machines, economic prosperity assured by resource depletion, and steady advancements in science and technology. Though most pay lip service to the teachings of their religious elders, the ethical and moral integrity of their inner, spiritual beliefs is usually offset by the struggle to survive the conditions of their outer worlds. It is a sorrowful thing for us to observe how humans have forgotten their true nature and purpose for living—that of God-seeking Souls who once freely danced along the interstellar webs.

Although the genetic pools from which starseeds' physical bodies are structured are usually biped mammalian, the essential nature—as it is for all beings—is that of Soul. The original starseeding took place much earlier than the rise of the mystical lands of Lemuria and Atlantis, and most Souls have long since lost the ability to remember antiquity's lost civilizations. But now their chakras are almost exploding with extrasolar energies, which awakening starseeds often interpret as kundalini events or supersexual orgasmic charges. Many are beginning to recall fragments of their Soul connectors to cosmic beings older than time itself.

Long ago, nuclei of omnipresent light journeyed to Earth from several star systems, among them Arcturus, the Pleiades, and Sirius. Surrendering to slumber, the original starseeds settled their energies into a variety of bodies to explore multiple species with a propensity toward intelligent evolution. In the early epochs of cooperative extrastellar Earth colonization, the star council's intent was to distill a variety of life-force energies onto the blossoming planet.

Many Arcturian starseeds were implanted on Earth five million years ago, when Cheuel was abruptly destroyed by its own inhabitants. Arcturian elders of the Crystal Blue Planet recognized the need for a planetary environment that presented Cheuelean Souls with unlimited opportunities to study the intricacies of Universal Law. Without further adieu they sent a colonization probe vessel to Earth.

By mutual agreement, the Cheueleans detached their Memory connectors to Arcturus. To assist them in their evolutionary journey, the Arcturian star council designed a system whereby the Cheueleans, after many lifetimes of experiencing an almost unlimited array of opportune Soul situations, would eventually balance the effects of the Law of Cause and Effect. They would then awaken to their Soul Memories when it came time for their new planetary mother, Earth, to ascend.

A few saintly souls from each of the Earth-seeding star systems agreed to retain Soul Memories in conscious awareness. Through the ages those enlightened beings have served humanity as master spiritual teachers. They are recorded in religious texts as avatars supreme, members of the great brotherhoods of light who keep silent surveillance over the Memories. Over the ensuing millions of years, the Dove of Peace, the Christed One, has kept vigilant watch over all slumbering starseeds, for Arcturus was certainly not unique in sending star probes to Earth. The finest effort of every human culture is to preserve and practice high holy teachings. Yet only the most advanced spiritually enlightened humans can equal in magnificence the beings of the brotherhoods of light. Eternally patient, the latter have long awaited starseed regeneration. Now the time has come for this generation to recognize that the perceived schism which separates them from the stars (and God) is an illusion. Starseeds are moving into the final stage of light-energy rejuvenation. As Earth poises for the last leg of her journey into the preludes of light-harmonics, her ascension into the refined dimension of the great galactic Home is near.

The Power of Thought

There exists within you a self-contained, emotional triage center, a place where exterior and interior impressions are gathered, sorted, recycled, and filtered into the appropriate brain compartment to be thoroughly considered and analyzed. Your most urgent thoughts, those that call for immediate attention, are situated at the forefront of your conscious thinking processes. Secondary thoughts take their places next in line, and so on, depending upon the degree of focused attention. The accumulated mental dynamics of a lifetime are absorbed and stored within the brain's neural centers. Thought is constantly on the move, one mental tidbit after another pushing its way into the forefront of the mind.

Brain gathers much of its information through physical input from the body's sense-gathering mechanics. Even so, acute eyesight is no guarantee of accurate internal perception. Even those with perfect vision cannot say that everything they observe about an event gives them a clear understanding of all its nuances. Sight, sound, taste, smell, feel—the sense organs cannot be judged completely trustworthy if the clarity of intuitive mind is not activated. The many substrates of external impressions cannot accurately serve a psyche that does not maintain a vigilant connection to Spirit.

When attention wanders into regions where ego-driven mental demons are at work, one retreats into the subtle and not-so-subtle areas of the personality's darker side. Mental scenarios continuously play out one drama after another, pulling attention away from Soul's efforts to maintain Itself, at all times, in a sublime state of higher Self alertness. Seemingly inconsequential, thoughts that grab the mind's attention are often the result of telepathic imprints instilled into the collective consciousness by the Dark Lords, whose primary interest is to control and manipulate mass human mind. Their primary weapon in the celestial tug of war, long waged in this galactic sector, is distraction. They perpetually try to cover the minds of sleeping humanity with a slimy ethereal substance that, once installed, insinuates itself throughout the brain and provides its host access to a delicious—to it—substance derived from fearful thought energies.

Although we urge you to defend yourself from these beings by an unwavering determination to contemplate peaceful, loving thoughts, we do not suggest you assume an anxious attitude of clenched-fingered, fitful prayer. Prayer and meditation are sacred devotional activities. We suggest you maintain a constant attitude of meditative prayer to achieve freedom from the incursions of negativity. As you reach levels of heightened spiritual awareness, you will eventually become immune to your ego and to unscrupulous beings. Meditation and prayer are essential activities for humans who are preparing for ascension.

Long ago, extraterrestrials came to Earth from the depths of several coarse-toned stars. In a rather willy-nilly fashion, those spiritually immature beings became attracted to newly forming Earth. In her youthful days, Earth shown like a beacon that drew dark beings like moths to a flame. A warp within the spatial filaments that separate vibrational densities was formed when the early populations of Sol-based planets, particularly Earth, Mars, and Maldek (whose violent demise created the asteroid belt that whirls between Mars and Jupiter), were pulled into a dubious alliance with dark beings. Thus, freewheeling beings from dingier atmospheric planes achieved Earth access. Their constant comings and goings climaxed in what could best be described as a celestial tug-of-war. The ongoing effect of this struggle—the negative disruption that has always plagued humans—is observable to even the most disinterested.

In the earliest of times, humans agreed to maintain themselves at a level of spiritual somnolence. This agreement is recorded in symbolic form as the fruit-and-serpent allegory in the Garden of Eden. Humans thus created a situation that accomplished little else than to fix their primary thoughts upon material acquisition. Certainly, the acquisition of objects is not the only goal of many people; however, it was practiced to such a high degree, particularly among the elite, that it created a race of myopic beings whose usual thought constructions were formed around ill-defined mental images.

To keep the multitudes of barely conscious humans from the grasp of negative entities requires massive cooperation from the angelic realms and the great brotherhoods of light. Poised to do battle, the angelic "armies" of the Archangel Michael and galactic beings pledged in service to the Office of the Christ have aligned themselves before Earth. Now the galaxy's perimeters are being restored to the harmonics of high-resolution light. Beware, for though the disrupters' game is over, more forceful remnants still remain who would gladly tease your Soul into joining them as they are transferred to another third-dimensional planet. In the evolutionary energies of the end times, humans who succumb to those entities are in imminent danger of destroying the finely tuned telepathic synapse responders buried within their midbrains.

To assist the newly aroused, crystalline implants are being inserted into their pituitary glands to prepare them for multidimensional telepathic exchange. Their thoughts have been energized by their primary guardians in conjunction with their higher Selves' permission and with special dispensation from the Office of the Christ. Although many remain telepathically untried, there is a growing sense within them that their minds are eagerly scanning the etheric strands for incoming messages. Few, however, have any real sense of the degree of their stimulated telepathic powers. Lacking substance, they continue to emit tentative thoughts that resemble the wispy feathers of a duckling. They have not yet discovered that their rapidly evolving minds have been equipped with all the mental tools they will need for extrastellar navigation.

The human mind is very much like a computer, constantly emitting, receiving, and storing waves of transmitted thought—most of it severely undisciplined. The human mind is naturally capable of telepathic communication with all beings via the galactically universal Language of the Sun. Unfortunately, humans' natural telepathic ability deteriorated from non-use, and they rest upon the planet like rusting cars. Batteries ebbing low, their minds emit feeble beeps now and then instead of the dynamic, pulsing, laserlike sparks for which their neural synapses were originally intended. We are supercharging those whose intention is to evolve spiritually. We jump-start the brains of those who call upon God to assist them. And a good jolt of telepathic energy will do them no harm.

That Which Calls Light to Earth is Omnipotent Wisdom. In service to That Which Is, the great brotherhoods of light have come together in cooperative Oneness to release this galactic outpost from the captive chains of the Dark Lords. We are sorting the wheat from the chaff, locating Souls who are responding to the quickening times in an enlightened and courageous manner. From out of the collective unconscious a few have traveled far enough along their spiritual paths to be capable of receiving high-intensity light. These mostly starseeded individuals are nearing the maximum in their efforts to regain Soul Memories. It is in service to them that we have retained the assistance of certain galactic beings whose membership in the star councils is recognized by their dedication to serve evolving Souls who reach Earth-graduate status. Their code, however, precludes interference without the human's conscious, willed request.

Those of you who are deeply sincere in your dedication to Spirit are reaching the moment when you will become telepathically active. Already you have freely and consciously formed a pact to work in cooperation with the galactic and angelic beings who have been assigned to facilitate your transposition to light.

Galactic Tools for Planetary Ascension

Like seas surging upon a rocky shore, Earth is being engulfed in waves of melodious spatial light and sound. As if raging water were washing over her, she is being wrapped in a deluge of uplifting cosmic energies. Perhaps, fair reader, as you reflect upon this statement you may feel entranced, as if you had stumbled upon a sacred mystery.

To make that which is obscure lucid, Malantor will further explain:

Beings of light who are assisting Earth's ascension into the light realms use exquisite light and luscious sound rays as adeptly as a skilled surgeon wields a scalpel to sever disease from an organ. Our crystalline energy rays are much less sharply plied than a physician's knife, however. We mingle harmonic tones (the music of the spheres) and exquisite colored light with naturally occurring cosmic energies that flow from Central Sun throughout the galaxy to create magnificent planetary sonatas. We use rays of singing light impregnated with the sweetest scents, as luxuriant as a bouquet of newly picked roses. Lustrous hues of radiant, scented, colored lights dance Earthward from our starships. We blend one colorful light strand with another to create a rainbow bridge effect over Earth.

Cosmic rays are the tools of our trade. To illustrate the manner in which light and sound become one, we will begin with the color red. Red is transferable to useful energy by vibrating it to the harmonic note C and mixing it with the scent of roses until the desired blend is achieved. Red has a powerful energy; it cleanses the land like lava from a volcano. Red has the ability to release a planet body's physical strain in the same way a surgeon operates upon injured tissues. Transformative red plunges deep into Earth, healing and penetrating her damaged organs. When red rays embrace Earth, her hum reverberates to note C and the air is alive with the scent of red, red roses.

Blue rays are abundant with the scent of dew-drenched bluebells and the hues of deep ocean water. Blue resonates with the melodious songs of dolphins and whales. Blue mirrors the vibrational tone of the Pleiades and resonates a color of emotional healing for Earth's sea creatures. Watery blue heals in a purifying manner in a way that fire does not. Watery blue covers the ashy residue of fire with special nutrients that are carried within it. Healing elements within watery blue restore hope in the hearts of animals and plants who live in water, just as a bright blue sky elevates the mood of land dwellers. Tranquil blue resonates to note G.

Yellow is used in many guises: pure yellow, yellow merging to orange, and yellow fading into a variety of browns, for yellow-to-brown earth tones are versatile. Yellow is the mustard seed, long a symbol for hope, trust, and faith. Yellow-yellow hums to the vibration of note E.

Yellow-orange wafts the scent of protective marigold, that lovely flower resembling our mother ship, *Marigold–City of Lights*. The melodious space cords delight in the yellow-orange hum, for golden yellow is the base harmonic of suns. Yellow-orange blends best with harmonic note D.

Yellow-brown hues are a reminder of the magnificent land masses. In the same way that mountains are solid, shades of yellow-orange-brown earth tones encourage emotional, mental, and physical stability. They resonate to notes D and E. Dark brown is the shade of dirt that harbors seeds and settles around the roots of plants and provides them with life-sustaining nutrients. Yellows, oranges, and browns signify loving protection for animals and plants. After the fiery reds and watery blues recede, the yellows, oranges, and browns remain to raise the qualities of the ground to higher-pitched vibration.

Green is the color of the tranquil, lush, floral Earth cover. Green resonates to note F, as does the heart chakra. Green is the tint of Earth Mother's gossamer, magical gown and the hue of her heart's deepest desires. Green emits essence of evergreen. Gigantic evergreens—redwoods, cedars, and pines—are guardians of Earth's lush forests. Green exhibits qualities of sturdy reliability, the knowledge that even the harsh cold of winter and the oppressive heat of summer cannot deter the evergreens from their vigilance over the forest floor. The seeds of evergreens are nurtured by the yellow-brown ground and are germinated by fire's red passion; their thirst is satisfied by flowing blue water. Green is the color of creative healing. Earth uses composites of green's vibration and refreshing odor to satisfy her need for creative expression.

If you lie close to Earth and stay very still, you will hear her softly humming. Her song resembles fluttering pine needles embraced by a soft breeze. Her natural vibration is the same as the outpouring of a human heart that is full with the joy of miraculous life.

Purple, violet, and indigo connect Earth to the spirit realms. They vibrate to notes A and B. Violet is the color of Earth's aura; it is her spiritual or essence vibration. Purples and violets are ripe with the scent of orchids. Fading to white, the lotus, the gardenia, the carnation, the space poppy, and all sweet flowers that exude white are gently tinged with violet. Purple to violet to white is symbolic of the delicate, transitory strength of flowers—one sweet color, one luscious odor, one gentle tone merging into the next. As the colors of flowers or of a rainbow naturally integrate one into the other, so the tone of A progresses into the vibrational pitch of B, and continues to C, D, E, F, and G, and then spirals into the resonation of a higher-octave A.

In worlds of light, there is no separation from Spirit as is perceived by humans. Dwelling in the heart of Love-Light Cosmic Mind, we experience all things as One. Etheric sound is one note—divine Aum—and spatial floral odor is one sweet fragrance. We do not fractionate this and that, and purple, like all colors, spans the entire cosmic spectrum.

Humans who work with color have as many viewpoints as there are people studying color, for each hue contains a multitude of properties. From a fifth- and sixth-dimensional perspective, that which is experienced as a particular note, hum, color, or odor is one and the same. If you were to organize everything humans have learned about light, color, sound, and odor and feed it into a computer for categorizing and analysis, on a third-dimensional level you would not be able to develop an understanding that the varying attributes of these things are parts of a whole. From our perspective, however, they are perceived as one quality essence.

In the upcoming years, a most delicious moment will transpire. It will be a moment of exquisite Divine Splendor. The clouds will melt into silver vapors and the oceans will resemble finely spun glass. Earth's physical elements will be elevated to the harmonics of Oneness that are indicative of the vibrational hum of the galactic core. All of Earth is now undergoing massive structural change. We are bombarding her with beams of light and sound that will eventually restore her youthful vigor.

Crop Circles and the Nature of Sacred Geometry

Statements included in this narrative are in accord with Patricia's particular mode of "channeling," her historical perspective, and her spiritual philosophy, and they may or may not reflect the opinions of others. She is a mystic, not a scientist. Keep in mind that while your anxious species has positioned telescopes to scan the doings of the universe, our observational ports are turned Earthward watching you. With this in mind, we begin.

Ley lines (also called Earth grids), crop circles, sacred geometry, and many ancient stone artifacts are reflected in the geometric forms of extrastellar starships. Particularly noteworthy as to their placement on Earth grids are Stonehenge, the Pyramid of Giza, Easter Island statues, and Mayan pyramids on the Yucatán peninsula–specifically Chichén Itzá, Palenque, and Uxmal. These edifices were formed from sacred geometrical patterns that are duplicated many times in alternate vibrational levels. To be more specific: The contours of Stonehenge and Avebury share equal energy patterns and are purposely positioned on Earth grids with the Pyramid of Giza. They are also geometrically aligned with both Atlantean and Lemurian temples, whose ancient foundations are buried beneath Easter Island and other Polynesian islands.

Many phenomenal Earth and extradimensional structures are being replicated symbolically in wheat-grass drawings popularly called crop circles. These mathematically correct displays of extrastellar art are not intended to last for more than a few days. In fact, many have a life span of but a few minutes, which humans often overlook.

Crop circles appearing in fields are formed from byproducts of naturally occurring geometry such as triangles, rectangles, and circles. Their structural math should not be looked upon as complicated, for if configured from the mathematics of music, their equations would be as simple as $1 + 1 = 2$. Their message will be missed if cosmic graphics are assumed to be difficult to correlate. Their symbolic meanings are intended to be understood by all people. Crop circles are tangible displays of sacred geometry. Not limited to this or that, some circles outline primary starship parameters, which are mirror images of the plants that cover Earth's green hills, which in turn are reflections of predominant extraterrestrial botanical species.

Subtly profound, these displays of sacred geometry are compatible with the discoveries of Pythagoras, Newton, and Einstein, and mathematical equivalents can be found in the music of Mozart. To limit Mozart to music and Pythagoras or Einstein (who are the same Soul) to the discipline of mathematics is to see complexity where none exists. We have previously suggested that the means to interstellar-multidimensional space flight is contained within the sacred geometric musical notes of Mozart's compositions. (This is an important clue for the evolution of humans into the greater galactic community.)

Sacred geometric shapes merge with and are duplicated in light, sound, and aroma. One is the other and the other is the One. All things in third-dimensional spatial time are reflections of atomic particles—geometric forms that duplicate whirling masses of stars called galaxies. Truly, that which is above is reflected in that which is below.

There is no hidden message in these data. We hope it is becoming obvious to those who have learned to think for themselves.

In addition to displays of multilevel sacred geometry and the power of the mathematics of music, many crop circles demonstrate the importance for humans to experience time as an extension of the intelligence of the One Mind. As long as they limit their spatial-time reference to a third-dimensional linear perspective, they will be unable to participate in galactic Now time. Now time is essentially circular. Many crop circles are attempting to communicate this important point.

It is a given: Geometric shapes are sacred. They are the material Prime Creator uses to form stars and planets, indeed, all matter. One of our many gifts to awakening humanity is the sacred symbol contained in crop circles. Crop circle formations are specifically designed to stir humans into accepting a broader-based reality. We suggest you look upon the circles thusly: Some simply illustrate that a rose is a rose is a rose, or that a musical note is a musical note is a musical note, or that a musical note is no different from a rose is a rose and that, in fact, a light prism is a light prism as well as a rose as well as a musical note. As multilevel light is sweetly scented, crop circles also illustrate that a star is a starship is a star.

Crop circles that represent flowers are designed around music as mathematical equations. Many are also symbolic representations of stone artifacts and the so-called gods and goddesses who came here aeons ago to starseed Earth. The impermanent nature of crop circles is a statement of the universal principle of ebb and flow, experienced in third-dimensional reality as birth-death or construct-destruct.

Crop circles as sacred geometry are expressions of sound, which is also light, which is also color, which is also aroma; they are expressions of universal vibration—the hum of the many planets. Crop circles are humanity's link to the stars. They are galactic teaching tools to help you gain a deeper understanding of the mathematics of music (vibration) and to assist you in detaching from your physical bodies so you can reactivate your light-bodies. This is a given.

Crop circles are mysterious only because you insist on viewing them as such. Crop circles are Pythagoras, they are atomic, they are Einstein, they are $E = mc^2$. Yes, they are quantum physics, but they are also a rose's blush and a laughing child. Crop circles outline the spiritual DNA of eagles, tigers, wolves, and whales. They fly, they crawl, they sing, they dance. Crop circle mathematical equations are equivalent to One, for they are representative of Omniscient Creator. Because of their sacred nature, they are formed of omnipotent Light-Love–Universal Intelligence.

Do not hinder your evolution to the stars by making complicated what is exquisitely simple. Sacred geometry is simply tonal vibration—combinations of Divine Light and Sound, the base material from which universes are birthed. As such, Light and Sound are components of crop circles as well as of pyramids and stone-faced statues staring up and down the corridors of Earth time.

It is recommended that these data be broken into their simplest components; that is, all forms of sacred geometry represent Love-Light in manifest reality.

Malantor for the Arcturian Council of Immaculate Light

Lemuria and Atlantis

Prior to the rising of the sea that created the great island continents of Lemuria (Mu, the Mother Land) and Atlantis, the world's land masses were in a perfect harmonious state of one. Lemuria was established prior to Atlantis by some thousands of years. Her inhabitants were direct descendants of starseeded individuals mainly from Andromeda, the Pleiades, Sirius, Arcturus, and Antares. From Andromeda the wee people came to peek from behind the ferns of lush, tropical Lemuria—so came the fairy people to Earth. From the Pleiades and Sirius telepathic whales and dolphins came to populate the seas. Long have these aware beings been in service to humanity. From Arcturus and Antares people of the light were placed to give service to their brothers and sisters planetwide, particularly to youthful, dynamic Atlantis.

Lemuria was originally established to prepare for an evolutionary technological event to occur when less-spiritually-structured Atlantis came into being. Her assignment was to stabilize and maintain Earth grids in a pattern of balanced light. In many ways, Earth herself was yet a youngster and prone to much restlessness; her tectonic plates were extremely active in those days. Lemurians also served the more physically oriented Atlanteans as spiritual nurturers, healers, advisors, and teachers. Lemurian-trained priests and priestesses were holders of light in Atlantean temples of worship.

Lemuria was home to a cross-section of starseeded saintly beings who built many fine cities and temples throughout her forests. Lemurian temples emitted such a purely refined energy that rainbows and glittering stardust swirled along the hallways and throughout all the rooms. Doorways were inscribed with sacred geometric designs—galactically inspired musical tones that are reemerging in today's crop circles. The golden doors were of such exquisite workmanship that they sang an individualized greeting to all who entered. Some allegorical tales of the time Earth was a Garden of Eden stem from Lemuria in her golden years.

Lemuria spanned a much greater area than is generally supposed. She stretched to what is now the U.S. Pacific Northwest, where her Eden-like gardens grew magnificent crystals as tall as pines. Psychics with the ability to peer into the fourth dimension can still see these giants. The Anasazi of the U.S. Southwest were Lemurian descendants. The Polynesians, Incas, and Easter Islanders were remnants from Lemurian civilizations. The faces of Easter Island were erected as Memory stones to capture the tears the people shed as their beloved motherland was swept away in a great deluge. Ever-watchful for the return of ships from the stars, the enigmatic stone faces stare at the sky from whence the star people are scheduled to return.

In harmony and peace Lemuria reigned for several thousand years before her rather rapid decline. In her latter years, she fell prey to the subtle yet powerful corrupting influence of her mated companion, technology-dominated Atlantis. Atlantis's brief spurt of glory gave the star councils much insight into the effects of unprecedented technological and scientific advancement in a species not yet mature enough to handle the ramifications of such wondrous things as time travel, nuclear energy, teleportation, and levitation. It soon became clear to them that to maintain the stability of the galactic core, Atlantis must fall.

Atlantis was home to the bawdy and the brave. Bright and cheerful in their youth—but tending toward bitterness in old age—the Atlanteans came to recognize that scientific knowledge in and of itself rings hollow in a spiritually unfulfilled race. The situation became grave when Lemuria lost her ability to steady the influx of mechanical genius with the balancing component of spiritual evolution.

When all was said and done, the Regency star council realized that the experiment in cooperatively aligning two diverse cultures on one planetary body was causing a schism directly affecting the tonal qualities of the planet's energy grids. Because of the direction in which technology's split from spirit was headed, the council voided the experimental colonization, intending to begin anew but at a slower pace that would allow time to blend all aspects of beingness within all the people. Thus, a great deluge and volcanic upheaval ripped apart Earth's continental plates. Breathing a great sigh, Lemuria and Atlantis slipped onto the ocean floor.

The Souls of Lemurians and Atlanteans, many having experienced multiple lives in both cultures, soon returned to third-dimensional life. About 10,000 B.C., present historical time, civilization reemerged at a slow, steady pace in the Tigris and Euphrates river valleys in Mesopotamia.

We end this limited view of Lemuria and Atlantis, civilizations whose existence is vehemently denied by modern-day archaeologists, historians, and scientists. Although that which is hidden is purposefully done, there is much evidence, if they but had the eyes to see farther than their noses point. To be fair to those passionate seekers of knowledge, evidence that is so compelling in legends is to be withheld from the masses until the end times. Humanity's haunting Soul Memories have kept not only Lemuria and Atlantis alive but also Camelot and many other fine tales that have warmed the human heart during history's long wintery night. As is spoken by the wise, "Where there is smoke, there is fire." Sagacious investigators are advised to make a deeper investigation into that which refuses to die.

Uncovering the Mysteries

To continue our dialogue on mysterious legends: As the years of change draw to a close, many things will surface that humans heretofore have not catalogued in textbooks. The Spiritual Hierarchy deliberately withholds prima facie evidence from starseeded planets until their inhabitants are mature enough to adequately assimilate it. Some cultures have shown greater potential for cosmic awareness than others. For instance, the Hopi (Hope-eee) people of the U.S. Southwest are among the clearest spatial-time prognosticators. Early Hopi visionaries accurately foretold interstellar fluctuations that would cause an unprecedented flow of transformative stellar energies around Earth. The Hopi and the Cherokee were two of many tribal peoples who ascertained the presence of solar energy grids we refer to as transdimensional universal intelligence—the system of ethereal lights that intergalactic starships use to glide from star to star. These grids are strands of vibrating light from which emanate the subtle odors of space poppies, roses, and lotuses. The streams of light strum in harmonic compliance with specialized hums (vibrations) of the solar bodies to which they are attached: suns or stars, planets, moons, comets, and so forth.

As the new century progresses, humanity is slated to experience an overt, multistar, multidimensional encounter. We do not mean to alarm you that Earth is to be overtaken by insectlike monsters. No indeed! We herald a most auspicious event. To prepare for this transformative moment, Earth is now [late 1990s] being inundated with successive waves of cosmic energy, which visionaries see as resulting from powerful fluctuating extrasolar winds.

The evolving elements of the Milky Way galaxy and her sister galaxies are spiraling upward upon filaments of corded lights that are redefining the vibrational hum of the entire multilevel universe. Souls resistant to change are pulling apart from Souls who have petitioned for ascension. The strain upon Earth's grids increases exponentially with the rate of restricted-thought attachment. As the positive and negative polarity increases, the strain intensifies, as if steel beams were about to buckle from a pressure buildup that far exceeds maximum tensile strength. It is obvious that at some point something will give.

The delicate colors, aromas, and tonal vibrations of the ethereal strands that connect Earth to the sun and other planets within the system will reach optimum tautness early in the new century. We will activate transmutation of blue sky to lavender-pink sky as the last remnant of tense-thought vibrations slough off this solar system's ethereal light cords.

As octave transmutation nears completion, the light cords will begin to flip, separate, divide, and regroup. For one brief micromoment, Earth will be cast free from the cords that bind her third-dimensional body to the solar grids before they are reconnected to cords that radiate refined light. For a blink of an eye, Earth and her inhabitants will be truly alone, for the strands that connect her lower dimensions to Divine Creative Impulse will completely sever. Immediately, she will slip through an upper-dimensional window where high-level strands will recapture her. Graduating Souls will meet their interstellar counterparts upon the starships. We will enfold their precious essences in a beatific net of unconditional Love. Thereafter, some Souls will opt to return to their heart-remembered starbase homes. Many quickening Souls, however, will wish to remain in Earth service until the new-dawn world is firmly established. Other valiant beings will elect to serve the nether worlds where beings reside in cosmic ignorance.

In these advancing years of the end times, we observe an intensification of natural and human-caused disasters. Modified by the unique happenstance of Earth's third-dimensional vibrations altering to fourth-degree status, in many subsurface regions tectonic plates are taking on a lustrous quality, as if made of porcelain instead of granite, limestone, and marble. Crustaceans and other creatures embedded in rock as the waters of ancient seas receded are not as dormant as may be supposed. Contrary to scientific rationalization, that which is dead and buried is not necessarily so. Eventually, as magma from newly forming volcanoes rises to the surface, long-buried crystalline structures holding Earth's true sacred and historical records will be uncovered.

We advise assayers, geologists, and gemologists—professionals trained in ascertaining qualities of diamonds and other precious stones—that a revision of carat count may be in order, a "higher" placement on your measuring scales, as it were. For instance, the angles of a gem mined in 1998, if carefully observed, would be noted to have a finer vibratory resonation than the angles of one mined in 1878, though the exterior of the gem would show no indication of being altered. Metallic substances such as gold, silver, and copper are evolving to the point that their atomic elements, as quantified by human standards, need to be redefined. What humans fail to take into account when measuring the atomic structures of metals and stones is the exquisite humming of their essences or anatomical-spiritual bodies.

Dear readers, and Patricia-Manitu as well, we do not wish to startle you with uneasy predictions that place you at the risk of looking foolish in the eyes of skeptics and intellectuals. We must reiterate, however, that most humans who study facts from solely a third-dimensional intellectual viewpoint fail to assimilate the prestigious teachings of the worlds' great spiritual leaders. They have always cautioned that the greatest truth is embedded in the words "Come and learn to practice compassionate, unconditional Love." Most do not even marginally understand that unconditional Love is an underlying universal force that naturally seeks to expand; that is, unconditional Love is evolutionary energy.

Mother Earth is a living being who is quite aware of the greater realities of Universal Law. As such, she is moving inexorably toward the day when she will no longer be trapped by the distressful boundaries of third-dimensional temporal law.

Those who care to pursue the wealth of information available that surely proves the existence of multidimensional starships must first contemplate the reason humanity's belief systems allow little room for the vibrational refinement of the material universe. It is imperative that humans begin to break down narrow, rigid thought systems to allow greater room for a universal spiritual cosmology.

Those who are without the faith of a mustard seed fail to heed this warning. Those bonded to outmoded religious and scientific notions are showing fearful signs of knee-jerk reflexes whenever they are approached with anything that hints of the paranormal. Those who view life narrowly fail to comprehend the broad universal scope of all things. Surely, they are in danger of missing the exquisite tides of evolutionary joy as the angels sing Earth's transformative song. As previously indicated, individual decision to evolve or not to evolve by applied, energetic, intentioned Will is the baseline criterion.

Reflections on the Phoenix Sightings

Popular sightings, those that stir the attention and imagination of the masses, often belong to the phenomenon of portal-shift opening. The 1997 sightings near Phoenix, Arizona, indicated a magnification of solar energies long prominent in that region, particularly in the Sedona area and around ancient Hopi and Navajo sacred sites. Intergalactic personnel are working principal Anasazi grid vortices. They are splicing solar-grid junction conduits in alignment with planetary grids, preparing for synergetic light-enhancement of the southwestern United States–northern Mexican starship corridor. The Luxor Hotel in Las Vegas, Nevada, being a mirror image of the Pyramid of Giza, is a vital resource tool for this work. The energy shield that was laid over the inhabitants of the southwestern United States–northern Mexican substrates in post-Lemurian times is now being lifted.

The Phoenix sightings, coupled with a proliferation of sightings in Mexico City over the last few years, are an indicator of third-dimensional energies yielding to fourth-dimensional configurations. Because of renewed interest by the Intergalactic Brotherhood of Light in these spatial regions, much activity—both extraterrestrial and terrestrial—is taking place in this vital area. Saucer- and triangular-shaped craft sighted in these geographic locations are often made on Earth with technology obtained from acquired extraterrestrial craft belonging to the Grays—with cooperation from them.

The activities of the Intergalactic Brotherhood are not limited to this area; we are preparing for the birthing of a world in Oneness. As such, Europe, Asia, Africa, Australia, South America, Canada, the North and South poles, and multiple island units are also engaged in temporal-to-etheric alignment. Even the deepest oceans are replete with images of visiting starships. Pleiadians and Sirians in particular are masters at water-grid logging and are busy plunging their ships into your watery depths. We who are Arcturians, among many others, prepare the ethers that surround Earth and the bulk of her continental plates with trajectories of light. Our light- and sound-enhanced tractor beams, which resemble crystalline lasers, are instrumental in transposing Earth from third-dimensional to etheric substance.

We suggest you become used to living with the wonderful sensation of accelerating grid power. You have only just begun to witness a proliferation of portal openings and the presence of illuminated disks, orbs, and multishaped starships that have long maintained silent residence in Earth's astral regions. Those who presume that we have newly come or that we mean to threaten and terrorize humanity should think again. We do not deny that there are deceitful extraterrestrials who are attempting to trick you into believing their motive is our motive as well. It will be your task, as you awaken to our presence, to discern which sightings and landings are ships that resonate Divine Light and which contain beings from the lower regions. As your superconscious Soul Memories download into your conscious minds, you will begin to recall when we mutually interacted, though it was a long, long time ago.

Do not the sacred books of all cultures hint of your brothers and sisters from the stars? What is so new? What is so quaint? What delays you is the presumption that you rein supreme in matters of universal intelligence. This is an old story, and it will soon be put to rest. Soon you will become much more enamored with your true natures—that of spiritual beings, cosmic inhabitants of a great star nation—than you are with your physical selves. Beings from the stars! Indeed. So are we. Thus are you!

Reflections on the El Niño Effect

In the precipitous climate of the late 1990s, an effect humans term *El Niño*, a symbolic representation of Christ-child energy, came upon the surface of the Earth, and a great deluge was upon the people. In His return through the portals of natural events, humans mistook the auspiciousness of the times as an act of God turned against them when, in fact, El Niño is an act of God turned in their favor. El Niño is a wake-up call, a call to return to a higher relationship with one another, all living creatures, and Mother Earth.

Earth, like a weeping mother who has amassed much misfortune at the hands of her children, is in the throes of a transformation. Therefore, El Niño may be correctly observed as Mother Earth shucking off her worn-out clothing for new vibrant garments. That which no longer serves her is leaving. That which is to her higher good is coming. El Niño represents an interim stage in Earth's evolutionary transition. Therefore, the process may best be observed as Divine in nature.

It is only fair, however, to take a critical look at the El Niño effect from the human standpoint. Of course, it is a time of mounting disaster. Is it not true that transformative events are often a point in life when a new way of perceiving raises one's focus to a higher state of consciousness? The ultimate goal of the Office of the Christ is to bring as many Souls Home as possible. Humans live in a dreamy vibrational substance. What they observe as solid and real is, in fact, as lacking in substance as dirt is when mixed with water to make a liquid mud. Water and wind are as necessary for Earth to cleanse herself as is a soapy bath to you.

For centuries, prophets have advised that there would be a reckoning for misusing planetary resources. Since the 1800s, Native American elders have made this quite clear. But technology-loving humans are becoming so self-absorbed that few look farther than their eyes can see. There have been intensifying signs of Earth changes for many years. Therefore, the El Niño effect should not come as a surprise. Nevertheless, the global-warming phenomenon continues to be perceived in many quarters as just that—a phenomenon, not an actuality.

We, too, have stated over and over that a reckoning is coming. Your leaders in particular are well aware of these things. Because seers have predicted these times for hundreds of years and modern-day prophets have been particularly verbose in their observations, why are so many questions raised of God when He, in fact, saw that you had adequate warning to prepare yourselves?

Weather is Earth's way of cleansing her body. Although this seems obvious to us, we are aware that it is not equally so from a third-dimensional standpoint. Therefore, we will outline a few details from a higher perspective. The celestial management team is assisting Earth to realign her anatomic structures to vibrate in harmony with fourth- and fifth-dimensional resonations. Our human co-workers, eagles of the new dawn, have been actively radiating thought forms of Love and Light into the planet's structural grids. They have been so successful that soon all fracture lines within the grid system will solidly realign. Our mutual endeavors have been instrumental in correcting an impending wobble that would have thrown Earth off her trajectory around the sun.

Earth's exterior body, her epidermis, is sloughing off old matter in much the same way your skin shakes off flakes of dead cells. It is as if Earth Mother is scratching herself to make herself more comfortable.

We do not wish to unduly alarm, but we do suggest that humans begin an all-out effort to overcome their fear of death and to learn to identify with themselves as Soul matter. Practical methods for achieving this sacred task are well outlined in many books.

As humans are evolving to less dense physical form so they may absorb and reflect light at the sublime level, plants and animals are also undergoing the same metamorphosis. In truth, the entire universe is at a genesis rebirth stage and resembles a flower bud about to open. A simultaneous upward and downward momentum is involved in this process—as if a flower were on top of another flower. The upper flower is about to loosen itself to set sail upon a breeze that will carry it into the sky of an alternate reality. The lower flower, however, is destined to drop to the ground, for it has chosen to continue its journey within the worlds of physical matter.

Animals are mirror images of humans. However, they are generally more alert than humans and their response to the quickening times is much faster. In actuality, many species are evolving right under your noses. Because humans are generally unable to view the long-term effects of a temporary anomaly, they tend to view animals' unusual antics, such as the increasing tendency of wild animals to enter humans' houses, as freaks of nature instead of as nature rhapsodizing herself on a higher-vibrational note. The rapidity of change is becoming so obvious that it will not be long before chameleonlike, adaptable humans slough off their old perceptions to make room for new.

Environmental changes such as pollution are certainly a reason for the accelerating numbers of animals and plants that are becoming extinct. What is not obvious, however, is that alert animals and plants are using these negative conditions to precipitate an exodus from Earth to return to their home worlds. Many reside in starship crystalline compartments awaiting the beginning of the beginning.

Many starseeded nonhuman species have come to love Earth deeply. They anxiously await her rejuvenation to light. After the beginning of the beginning, they will opt to return. To facilitate their free-will choices, a business meeting with humans via the auspices of the Regency star council will take place. They will mutually agree to dwell together in an Eden-like environment upon a renewed Earth. From a higher-dimensional perspective, this is already a fait accompli, and the proceedings will be only a formality.

It is imperative that humans learn to think of Earth as a vital, living being. From a Soul standpoint, it is of little benefit to become frantic over Earth changes. Earth Mother is simply a reflection of your latent abilities to transform yourselves into mature-state beings. But you are not even aware that your thoughts are so powerful they have directly contributed to the situation you now find yourselves in. You are so fearful of acknowledging your ability to cocreate with higher-dimensional beings of light! When you do so, you will indeed be One in harmonic rapture with us, a state of being that knows no separation between itself and all aspects of Creation. Then you will understand what life is really about!

Lest it escape your notice, prophecies for the sinking of California into the Pacific Ocean have been softened. Because of the good works of humans who have spent many years sending loving, healing thoughts to Earth, that which had long been foreseen has not occurred. Is it not true that California is now underwater—but in a much gentler fashion? Is this not cause for much celebration?

Returning Home

Life's difficulties are temporarily forgotten by those who direct their attention to physical pleasure when their sorrow and pain become too intense. Now, for those of you who are awakening, your Soul Memories are beginning to slide into conscious awareness. Many of you long to escape Earth's confines, to return Home. Like a beacon shining through a stormy night, the brilliant light of Greater Home, Central Sun, lights your way while it summons your Souls.

Many seek refuge from the stresses of daily life. The often harsh realities of human society weigh heavy upon your slumbering Souls. Sorrow spent, your day will come. You who are evolving will one day lift off like eagles on the wing. Your physical forms will turn to light, your minds will flush clean all vestiges of karmic debris, and your spirit bodies will shine like the noonday sun. As blissful light pours through your every cell, you will mount the wings of Spirit. In ecstasy you will dance with beings of light who drift along the ethereal stargrids.

Embrace the dream that heart-minded humans of all ages have always dreamed. The Milky Way, long denied you, will soon open the golden-portaled pathway that leads to Celestial Home. Interstellar flight, long humanity's dream, is about to be yours. Yours!

"What! Me?" you cry. "Me?" Indeed, that which is ours is also to be yours. That which is dormant within you is about to give birth to new form. Like a wee bird emerging from its shell, you are pecking and pecking your determined way to freedom. You are about to hatch the stars. Do you hear your Soul crying to you to come Home? "Come Home little bird, come Home! Return to the light." You, all eagerness and joy, are mounting a stairway that will open upon an illustrious platform of God-realized enlightenment. Your long Soul struggle, the effort it has taken to crawl out from the ooze to the realities of higher-dimensional light, is almost done. You have spent uncounted lifetimes in your course to regain the stars.

As you are becoming aware that you are about to access the space grids, your feelings of entrapment are intensifying. Frustrated, you petition your celestial guides to hurry, hurry, hurry. You urge them to take you up in their beatific arms and carry you safely away. But not yet, not yet. There are things awaiting, tasks that need completing, a few final feathers to discard before lightness of being and permanent liftoff can be accomplished.

Wish for Home, to return to the stars, to the hallways of God's Peaceful Portals. Wish for it with all your might. Desire it above all things.

To help you prepare for this awesome journey, we encourage you to take a preview glimpse by meditating and envisioning yourself exploring Mars, Venus, and the moon Eros. Without fear, dive into Jupiter's fiery depths. Become one with Saturn's humming crystalline rings as they drift around her. Place yourself before rosy Arcturus, Andromeda, Sirius, Antares, and the seven sisters of the Pleiades. Look far, far into the stellar distances that only mystical dreamers are able to see. Imagine being as light as a feather and lighter still until the sensations of your physical body momentarily disappear. Know you are One with all things, that you are held in the Omniscient Mind of Source Creator. Now you are already Home. You are a nebula. You are a birthing star. You are a glorious birthing universe!

This is you! This is us-we-you as well!

You have always been a star traveler. You have always been a being of infinite light. No longer allow the situation of being human to tell you differently. Unfurl your angel wings and mount the podium of cosmic awareness that will jettison you to the stars. Home, Home to stay.

Malantor–Words of Summation

Now that you have studied the far-reaching data in this extraterrestrial manuscript, the vibrations of their renderings may trigger within your brain-mind previously dormant abilities and Soul Memories. As you continue your journey to the higher realms, daily contact with higher Self's presence will become an ecstatic reality.

Transcripts contained in this volume of the Arcturian Star Chronicles are a cooperative, coordinated effort between Patricia-Manitu of planet Earth and Malantor, a light-essence Arcturian being and a member of the Intergalactic Brotherhood of Light Regency star council. Upper-dimensional extraterrestrials who knock at the doors of awakening humans' conscious minds maintain themselves at all times in parallel energy alignment with the Spiritual Hierarchy and Source Creator. Telepathic wavelengths transmitted by Arcturians through Patricia are designed to intensify humans' awareness of Universal Law and their greater galactic family. Arcturians and other higher-dimensional extraterrestrials act in accord with orchestrations of the celestial hum that is Essence of the Christ.

To aid in your appreciation of how we are attempting to communicate with you personally, we would have you understand how we gather thoughts and deposit them in crystalline "computer" starship monitoring stations. Because verbal speech is inherently limiting and incapable of accessing the rich purity of telepathic communication, human mental constructions are initially filtered through the sun, where their configurations are restructured into tonal qualities of the universally understood solar language. The sun's solar library filters out thought impurities so that the full essence of truth underlying any thought is fully integrated before being transposed intact to our crystalline monitors. That is, the intentions of your intuitive heart-mind and your logical brain-mind are reduced to the delicate fabric of their innate properties. Then they are handed off, as it were, to the light-entity who serves you in the capacity of guidance counselor or spiritual guardian. Solar language, at all times, is in harmonic agreement with One, with Divine Mind. Thus, communication at this level is always in alignment with the dynamic rhythms of higher-octave Galactic Mind.

You are cautioned, gentle reader: The solar resource library (which is available to all awakening life forms, not only humans) must never be used for recreational or thrill-seeking purposes. Like leaves dropping from autumn trees, such enticements will cause your precious thoughts to become like starship dust, and they will be swept into the lower realms or astral oblivion.

Though the energies of this manuscript fade, Malantor has only begun to speak. As the bonnet of Earth's future is securely tied, we who dwell in starships will remain vigilant to protect her. May you who possess clarity of vision remain acutely aware of our presence and our purpose for being here.

From our glorious starship *Marigold–City of Lights*, Malantor's energies become quiescent. This day of days that sees the completion of Malantor's transmissions also heralds their beginnings, for I am to return with others of my kind to puncture the last vestiges of enduring pain that hold your wounded hearts captive. We will open eternity's golden doors before your wondering eyes. For you who already travel embedded in your Souls' womb, starship portals stand open and ready to receive you.

Adonai to you, most gracious reader.

Malantor's Concluding Songs

From out of the depths of starless nights I come.
From out of a murky abyss where dark oceans failed
    to capture the light of a noonday sun.
Arousing from my restless slumber, I became Malantor,
    a being of eternal, essential light.
In my Soul travels I have been witness to the birthing
    of untried universes.
Gifted, as are all beings, by Divine Creator
    with the ability to become,
I have discovered the Oneness of Being from which
    stars are formed.

Capture this vision and set it free.
Capture its spirit and you, too, will come to know
    the manifestations of Perfect Love
        that merciful God grants to all Its creation.

In Grace you become still,
In Love you become serenely at peace.
Calm as water flowing over submerged rocks,
Stately as the tallest tree,
That which awakens within you is a consequence of
becoming attuned to Earth's evolving rhythms.
As you learn to solidly concur with spiritual guidance,
you will become One with all universal beings.
Are you not aware you are being shown the way Home?

Refreshing, never daunted, spiritually activated Souls
swarm around Earth like bees searching for
honeyed flowers.
Is nectar of sweet ambrosial nirvana known in our realms?
Indeed it is.
Seek that.
All else follows.
Omniscient, Omnipotent Creator is your closest ally
in the greatest moment Earth's inhabitants have ever
known: a return to the stars.
Envision this now!

Appendix

Glossary

ADONAI: Hebrew for "Lord." Divine energy associated with the word's vibration assures Patricia of her light-level telepathic connection.

AKASHIC RECORDS: Cosmic journals that contain the records of the Soul's journey. These records are attended to by the angelic realms. With permission, Earth's spiritual masters and empowered enlightened beings are able to peruse the records.

ASCENDED MASTERS: Earth-incarnated souls who have overcome death, have assumed their bodies of light, and have attained God-realized Christ Consciousness.

ASTRAL PLANES: Fourth dimension, planes of instant manifestation. The astral is where reincarnating souls attached to Earth dwell between lives. The astral planes are vast and multilayered. The lower astral is where negative beings and negative thought forms reside. The region referred to in religious texts as heaven is the upper astral. See *Octave*.

Aum, Ohm: Prime tone, a basic ingredient of universal energy. See *Hum*.

Blue Crystal Planet: Closest English translation for the principal light-body planet of the Arcturian star system. Primary planning and gathering planet for the multiuniversal, multidimensional star councils.

Brain-mind: The logical mind where the computerlike calculations of the physical brain are stored. See *Conscious mind, Heart-mind, Subconscious mind,* and *Superconscious mind.*

Brotherhoods of light: Brotherhood means *in Oneness*. There are many orders of brotherhoods of light. Earth's embodied and ascended masters are members of these brotherhoods. The Intergalactic Brotherhood of Light, which is made up of spiritually advanced extraterrestrials, is one order. Another important brotherhood associated with Earth's ascension is the Order of Melchizedek. The Office of the Christ heads the brotherhoods of light. *The Book of Knowledge: The Keys of Enoch* by J. J. Hurtak is an excellent resource for information on the brotherhoods. See "Suggested Books and Movies." See *Intergalactic Brotherhood of Light.*

Celestial Home: Also referred to as Central Sun. The Soul yearns to return to Celestial Home. It is the Soul's journey's end.

Cellular matrices: The molecular makeup of all third-dimensional physical matter. Used to describe the human body as well as Earth's body.

CHAKRA: Wheels of energy that make up the body's inner anatomy. Often described as lotus blossoms in Eastern tradition. Chakras are widely covered in Hindu, Buddhist, and Yoga texts. Shirley MacLaine's "Inner Workout" video is an excellent study and meditation source for the Western mind.

CONSCIOUS MIND: Third-dimensional brain functions. Mental layers of linear-logical thought. Same as brain-mind. See *Brain-mind, Heart-mind, Subconscious mind,* and *Superconscious mind.*

DARK LORDS: Evil, manipulative, controlling beings who throughout history have attempted to hold humanity in their clutches. They are referred to as satanic beings, Lucifer, and the dark angels. See *Grays.*

DENSITY OCTAVE, DIMENSIONAL OCTAVE: See *Octave.*

EAGLES OF THE NEW DAWN: Awakened humans (and animals) who interact with the star councils to serve Earth's evolution. Also called sky warriors.

ENERGY FIELDS: Energy fields range from subtle to force-field magnitude. The energy field that surrounds the human body is the aura. See *Grids* and *Vortex.*

ETHERIC GRID STRANDS: See *Grids.*

FIFTH DIMENSION: Dimension of refined light. Arcturians are fifth- and sixth-dimensional beings. Negative beings are unable to penetrate into the realms of light substance.

FOURTH DIMENSION: See *Astral planes.*

GOD-REALIZED: An enlightened, evolved individual who has attained Christ Consciousness. Spiritual masters are God-realized.

GRACE: To receive grace is to be held in the fluttering arms of angels. Grace is an energy field that descends upon humans from Divine sources for physical, emotional, and mental healing, and to assist in fulfilling the Soul's life purpose.

GRAYS: Manipulative extraterrestrials who are in alliance with the Dark Lords. The Grays are responsible for human abductions and cattle mutilations. See *Dark Lords*. See *Hidden Mysteries* by Joshua D. Stone and *UFOs and the Nature of Reality* from Ramtha for detailed information.

GRIDS, GRIDLINES, SPACE GRIDS, STARGRIDS, STRANDS: Crisscrossing webs of light, sound, color, and scent that make up Earth's spiritual body. Starships also travel upon grids of light that weave through space. Grids of light connect galaxy to galaxy, star to star, planet to planet, moon to moon, and so forth. Refer to Volume I, Part III for more detailed information.

HARMONIC COORDINATES OF THE GALACTIC HUM: The sound coordinates of the grids. See *Hum*.

HEART-MIND: The intuitive, spiritual mind. The heart chakra is the location of the heart-mind. It is where we connect with our higher Selves and our Soul Memories. See *Brain-mind*, *Conscious mind*, *Subconscious mind*, and *Superconscious mind*.

HUM: Cosmic creative vibration, the prime or God energy expressed as Aum (Amen) or Ohm. Matter's tonal qualities. Pythagoras described hum as the music of the spheres.

I AM: The Self's identity as Soul.

Intergalactic Brotherhood of Light: Spiritually evolved, light-formed, fifth- and sixth-dimensional extraterrestrials from many star systems and many universes. See *Spiritual Hierarchy* and *Star councils.*

Language of the Sun: Common mode of telepathic communication natural to all beings. Also called solar tongue or solar language.

Light-Love or Love-Light: Light is the first manifestation of God in form; Love is God's Essence or energy. Light-Love incorporates Creation's energy as a physical manifestation. Sound (vibration) is integral to Light-Love energy. Throughout the ages Earth's God-realized spiritual masters have referred to Light-Love as unconditional Love.

Light strands: See *Grids.*

Lords of Darkness: See *Dark Lords.*

Love and love: Unconditional Love is integrated Cosmic Intelligence. However, love is the emotion humans feel for others, their pets, and Earth.

Manitu: Meaning "spirit keeper," it is the title the Intergalactic Brotherhood bestows on people whose life's purpose is planetary healing.

Marigold–City of Lights: Intergalactic Brotherhood Earth-based mother ship. Authors may refer to it by other names, perhaps *City of Lights*, *Jeweled City*, *Crystal City*, *New Jerusalem.* The term *Marigold* was given to this writer as a symbolic clue that cosmic light incorporates vibration, color, and scent. The mother ship in the movie *Close Encounters of the Third Kind* portrays her essence, though *Marigold–City of Lights* is much larger.

MEMORIES: Aspect of Self-knowledge slumbering humanity has forgotten; Soul Memories. As we awaken to our spiritual nature, the Memories are reactivated.

OCTAVE: A dimensional or density span. The vibrational layers within a dimension are not unlike the notes of the musical scale, ever softening in an upward or refining manner.

PSYCHIC PROTECTION: The purposeful use of Light-Love when meditating or channeling. The following steps are recommended: cleansing one's physical environment with incense or sacred herbs (smudging); requesting Christ Consciousness energy (see *Spiritual Hierarchy*) to assist; visualizing light running through the chakras and surrounding the body in an energy bubble; using a repetitive, vibrational tone or mantra (for example, Aum or Ohm); and routinely forcefully challenging any entity with the statement "Are you of the Light (spiritual beings)?" (See Volume I, Part II, "Patricia Meets Palpae.") Beings of light expect to be challenged. Negative beings cannot penetrate the layers of a Light-Love established forcefield.

RESONANT VIBRATIONAL HUM: Degree of refined light vibrating within a dimensional octave.

SIXTH DIMENSION: See *Fifth dimension.*

SKY WARRIORS: See *Eagles of the new dawn.*

SPACE GRIDS: See *Grids.*

SPACE POPPIES: Refers to scented, flowered coordinates that are the by-products or the bouquets of the harmonics. The Arcturians find the symbolic use of flowers helpful in explaining the fragrant qualities of the light grids.

SPACE-TIME: In this text, refers to the linear structures of third-dimensional spatial and time realities as well as to the ebb and flow of fourth-dimensional space and time.

SPIRITUAL HIERARCHY: Body of One, supreme spiritual council in service to Earth's ascension. The central figure is the Christ Essence. The council includes archangels and angelic realms, ascended masters, the brotherhoods of light (including the Intergalactic Brotherhood of Light), and God-realized humans.

STAR COUNCILS: Coordinators and directors of multispatial, intergalactic business affairs. All aware galactic citizens have input upon the star councils. Arcturians in service to Earth sit upon the star councils as a subdivision of the Supreme Hierarchical Council for Planetary Ascension, System Sol, Intergalactic Brotherhood of Light.

STAR GRIDS: See *Grids*.

STARGATE: A multidimensional access window. See the movies *2001: A Space Odyssey* and *Stargate* for a graphic portrayal of stargate dynamics.

STARSEEDS: Galactic beings on Earth as humans, animals, and plants. Many universes and star systems are represented, among them Arcturus, Pleiades, Sirius, and Orion.

STRANDS: See *Grids*.

Subconscious mind: The spirit-mind, or intuitive heart-mind, that receives information from the superconscious, transforms it into symbols the brain-mind can understand, and then sends it to the brain-mind, or conscious mind. See *Brain-mind, Conscious mind, Heart-mind*, and *Superconscious mind.*

Superconscious mind: Soul mind, or higher Self mind. It uses the subconscious mind as a conduit to send information to the brain-mind, or conscious mind. See *Brain-mind, Conscious mind, Heart-mind*, and *Superconscious mind.*

Universal Law: The Law of One. One song (for) all.

Vortex: Varying degrees of heightened energies that arise from a point along a grid where light strands crisscross. Vibration and light energy arising from a vortex varies greatly and may range from a few inches to miles. Intuitively, humans have always recognized vortices as power spots or sacred sites. Refer to Volume I, Part III for more detailed information.

Yin-yang: Ancient Chinese symbol used in the teachings of the Tao and the I Ching. Yin is feminine; yang is masculine. Yin-yang demonstrates all polarities and diversities (the ten thousand things) that exist within the universal whole.

Suggested Books and Movies

Books

Agartha: A Journey to the Stars. Meredith Lady Young-Sowers. Walpole, N.H.: Stillpoint, 1984.

Alchemy of the Human Spirit: A Guide to Human Transition into the New Age. Kryon (Spirit), [channelled by] Lee Carroll. Del Mar, Calif.: Kryon Writings, 1996.

Aliens Among Us. Ruth Shick Montgomery. New York: Fawcett, Crest, 1985.

An Act of Faith: Transmissions from the Pleiades. P'taah (Spirit), [channelled by] Jani King. The P'taah Tapes series. Cairns, Queensland, Australia: Triad, 1991; York Beach, Maine: Samuel Weiser, 1996.

Ancient America. Jonathan Norton Leonard. Great Ages of Man; A History of the World's Cultures series. (Nazca Lines.) New York: Time-Life Books, 1967.

Arcturus Probe. José Argüelles. Sedona, Ariz.: Light Technology Communication Services, 1996.

Autobiography of a Yogi. Paramahansa Yogananda. Los Angeles: Self-Realization Fellowship, 1946.

Bashar: Blueprint for Change: A Message from Our Future. Bashar (Spirit), [channelled by] Darryl Anka. Edited by Luana Ewing. Seattle: New Solutions, 1990.

Beyond Ascension. Joshua D. Stone. Sedona, Ariz.: Light Technology Communication Services, 1995.

Beyond Stonehenge. Gerald S. Hawkins. New York: Harper & Row, 1973; New York: Marboro Books, Dorset, 1989.

The Book of Knowledge: The Keys of Enoch. J. J. Hurtak. Los Gatos, Calif.: Academy for Future Science, 1977.

Bringers of the Dawn: Teachings from the Pleiadians. Barbara Marciniak. Santa Fe, N.M.: Bear, 1992.

Celestial Raise: 'Tiers of Light' Pouring Fourth from the Son. Edited by Marcus. Mt. Shasta, Calif.: ASSK (Association of Sananda and Sanat Kumara), 1986.

Circular Evidence: A Detailed Investigation of the Flattened Swirled Crops Phenomenon. Pat Delgado and Colin Andrews. Grand Rapids, Mich.: Phanes Press, 1989.

The Complete Ascension Manual for the Aquarian Age. Joshua D. Stone. Sedona, Ariz.: Light Technology Communication Services, 1994.

The Cosmic Connection: Worldwide Crop Formations and ET Contacts. Michael Hesemann. Bath, England: Gateway Books, 1996.

The Crystal Stair: A Guide to the Ascension: Channeled Messages from Sananda (Jesus), Ashtar, Archangel Michael, and St. Germain. Eric Klein. Edited by Sara Benjamin-Rhodes. Livermore, Calif.: Oughten House, 1990; third edition, 1994.

The Divine Romance. Paramahansa Yogananda. Los Angeles: Self-Realization Fellowship, 1986.

Don't Think Like a Human!: Channelled Answers to Basic Questions. Kryon (Spirit), [channelled by] Lee Carroll. Del Mar, Calif.: Kryon Writings, 1994.

The Earth Chronicles series. Vols. I–V. Zecharia Sitchin. New York: Avon Books; Santa Fe, N.M.: Bear, 1980–1993.

Earth's Birth Changes. St. Germain (Spirit), [channelled by] Azena Ramada. St. Germain Series. Cairns, Queensland, Australia: Triad; York Beach, Maine: Samuel Weiser, 1996.

The End Times, New Information for Personal Peace: Channelled Teachings Given in Love. Kryon (Spirit), [channelled by] Lee Carroll. Del Mar, Calif.: Kryon Writings, 1992.

E.T. 101: The Cosmic Instruction Manual for Planetary Evolution. Mission Control (Spirit), [channelled by] Zoev Jho. San Francisco: HarperSanFrancisco, 1994. Originally published as channelled by Diana Luppi (1990).

The Findhorn Garden. Findhorn Foundation. New York: HarperCollins, 1975.

God I Am: Inspired by the Triad of Isis, Immanuel and St. Germain. Peter O. Erbe. Cairns, Queensland, Australia: Triad; York Beach, Maine: Samuel Weiser, 1996.

The Gods of Eden: A New Look at Human History. William Bramley. New York: Avon Books, 1989.

Hidden Mysteries. Joshua D. Stone. Sedona, Ariz.: Light Technology Communication Services, 1995.

Lazaris (Spirit) series books, videos, and cassettes. Palm Beach, Fla.: Visionary Publishing.

Life and Teachings of the Masters of the Far East. Vols. I–V. Baird T. Spalding. Marina del Rey, Calif.: DeVorss, 1924.

Mary's Message to the World: As Sent by Mary, the Mother of Jesus, to Her Messenger Annie Kirkwood. Mary, Blessed Virgin, Saint (Spirit), [channelled by] Annie Kirkwood. Edited by Brian Kirkwood. New York: Putnam, 1991; New York: Berkley, Perigee, 1996.

The Mayan Factor: Path Beyond Technology. José Argüelles. Santa Fe, N.M.: Bear, 1987.

The Monuments of Mars: A City on the Edge of Forever (book and video). Richard C. Hoagland. Berkeley, Calif.: North Atlantic Books, Frog, Ltd., 1987.

The Nature of Personal Reality: Specific, Practical Techniques for Solving Everyday Problems and Enriching the Life You Know (and other Seth series books). Seth (Spirit), [channelled by] Jane Roberts. Englewood Cliffs, N.J.: Prentice-Hall, 1974; San Rafael, Calif.: Amber-Allen, 1994.

Nothing in This Book Is True, But It's Exactly How Things Are: The Esoteric Meaning of the Monuments on Mars. Bob Frissell. Berkeley, Calif.: North Atlantic Books, Frog, Ltd., 1994.

The Only Planet of Choice: Essential Briefings from Deep Space. Phyllis V. Schlemmer. Edited by Mary Bennett. Bath, England: Gateway Books, 1993; revised edition, 1996.

A Path with Heart: A Guide through the Perils and Promises of Spiritual Life. Jack Kornfield. New York: Bantam Books, 1993.

The Pleiadian Agenda: A New Cosmology for the Age of Light. Barbara Hand Clow. Santa Fe, N.M.: Bear, 1995.

Project World Evacuation: UFOs to Assist in the "Great Exodus" of Human Souls off this Planet. Compiled through Tuella by the Ashtar Command. Edited by Timothy Green Beckley. Petaluma, Calif.: Inner Light Publications, 1993.

Ramtha. Ramtha (Spirit), [channelled by] J. Z. Knight. Edited by Steven L. Weinberg. Eastsound, Wash.: Sovereignty, 1986.

The Sirius Connection: Unlocking the Secrets of Ancient Egypt. Murry Hope. Rockpart, Mass.: Element Books, 1996.

Something in This Book Is True–. Bob Frissell. Berkeley, Calif.: North Atlantic Books, Frog, Ltd., 1997.

The Star-Borne: A Remembrance for the Awakened Ones. Solara. Charlottesville, Va.: Star-Borne, 1989.

The Starseed Transmissions. Ken Carey. San Francisco: HarperSanFrancisco, 1991.

Surfers of the Zuvuya: Tales of Interdimensional Travel. José Argüelles. Santa Fe, N.M.: Bear, 1988.

The Third Millennium: Living in the Posthistoric World. Ken Carey. San Francisco: HarperSanFrancisco, 1995. Originally published as *Starseed, the Third Millennium* (1991).

The Tibetan Book of Living and Dying: A New Spiritual Classic from One of the Foremost Interpreters of Tibetan Buddhism to the West. Sogyal Rinpoche. San Francisco: HarperSanFrancisco, 1993.

Transformation of the Species: Transmissions from the Pleiades. Jani King. The P'taah Tapes series. Cairns, Queensland, Australia: Triad.

The Treasure of El Dorado: Featuring "the Dawn Breakers." Joseph Whitfield. Roanoke, Va.: Treasure, 1977; reprint, 1989.

UFOs and the Nature of Reality: Understanding Alien Consciousness and Interdimensional Mind. Ramtha (Spirit), [channelled by] J. Z. Knight. Edited by Judi Pope Koteen. Eastsound, Wash.: Indelible Ink, 1990.

We, the Arcturians. Norma J. Milanovich. Albuquerque, N.M.: Athena, 1990.

With Wings As Eagles: Discovering the Master Teacher in the Secret School Within. John R. Price. Boerne, Texas: Quartus Books, 1987; Carson, Calif.: Hay House, 1997.

You Are Becoming a Galactic Human. Washta (Spirit), [channelled by] Virginia Essene and Sheldon Nidle. Santa Clara, Calif.: SEE (Spiritual Education Endeavors), 1994.

MOVIES ("MANAGEMENT TRAINING FILMS")

2001: A Space Odyssey. Stanley Kubrick film.

2010: The Year We Make Contact. Peter Hyams film.

Abyss. James Cameron film.

Always. Steven Spielberg film.

Batteries Not Included. Steven Spielberg film.

Close Encounters of the Third Kind (extended version). Steven Spielberg film.

Cocoon. Ron Howard film.

Contact. Robert Zemeckis film.

Defending Your Life. Geffen Pictures.

Field of Dreams. P. A. Robinson film.

Ghost. Jerry Zucker film.

Heart and Souls. Ron Underwood film.

Heaven Can Wait. Paramount.

Hoagland's Mars. Richard C. Hoagland.

Made in Heaven. Lorimar Motion Pictures.

Phenomenon. Touchstone Pictures.

Planetary Traveler. Third Planet Entertainment.

Powder. Hollywood Pictures.

Shirley MacLaine's Inner Workout. High Ridge Productions.

Star Trek (entire series, both motion pictures and television, especially *Star Trek IV: The Voyage Home*).

Star Wars trilogy: *Star Wars, The Empire Strikes Back, Return of the Jedi.* George Lucus films.

Stargate. Mario Kassar film.

Starman. John Carpenter film.

Willow. Ron Howard film.

Beyond Words Publishing, Inc.

OUR CORPORATE MISSION:

Inspire to Integrity

OUR DECLARED VALUES:

We give to all of life as life has given us.

We honor all relationships.

Trust and stewardship are integral to fulfilling dreams.

Collaboration is essential to create miracles.

Creativity and aesthetics nourish the soul.

Unlimited thinking is fundamental.

Living your passion is vital.

Joy and humor open our hearts to growth.

It is important to remind ourselves of love.

Printed in the United States
By Bookmasters